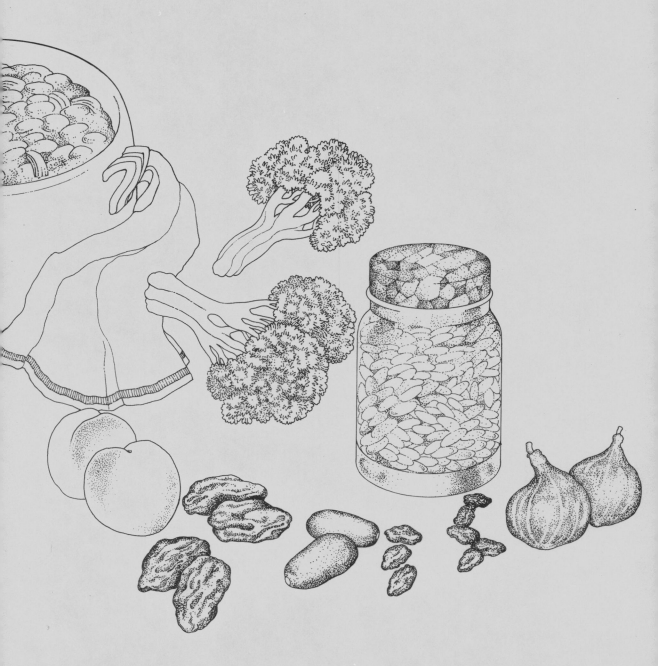

100 High Fibre Dishes

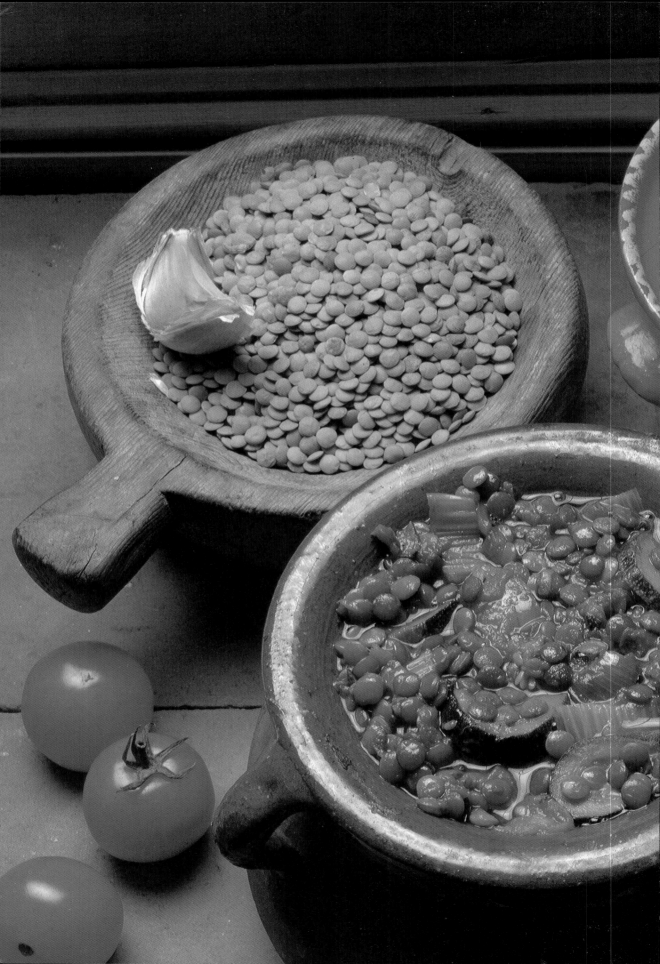

100
High Fibre Dishes

Edited by
Jenni Taylor

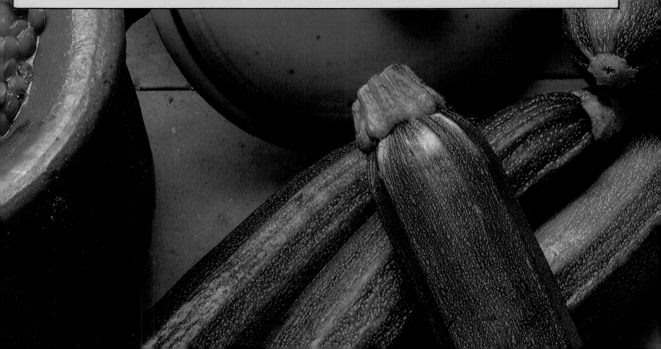

octopus

Contents

Notes
Standard spoon measurements are used in all recipes
1 tablespoon = one 15 ml spoon
1 teaspoon = one 5 ml spoon
All spoon measures are level

Fresh herbs are used unless otherwise stated.
Where amounts of salt and pepper are not specified, the cook's discretion should be used when adjusting the seasoning.
Ovens and grills (broilers) should be preheated to the specified temperature or heat setting.
For all recipes, quantities are given in metric, imperial and American measures. Follow one set of measures only, because they are not interchangeable.

First published 1984 by
Octopus Books Limited
59 Grosvenor Street, London W1

© 1984 Octopus Books Limited
ISBN 0 7064 2054 3
Produced by Mandarin Publishers Ltd
22a Westlands Road
Quarry Bay, Hong Kong

Frontispiece: Mediterranean Lentil Stew (page 16)

Introduction

Dietary fibre is receiving an ever increasing amount of publicity and it is now considered to be an essential part of our daily diet. But what is dietary fibre? It used to be known as roughage and is mainly the indigestible rigid material from which plant cell walls are made.

Because of its indigestibility food manufacturers in the Western World tend to remove it during the processing or refining of foods. This is particularly true in the processing of wheat. Bran, the outer fibrous layer or husk of the wheat, is removed to produce white flour which in turn is used in the production of many flour based foods including bread, pasta, cakes and biscuits.

The medical profession is of the opinion that it is our highly refined diet that contributes to the high increase in incidence of diseases related to the digestive tract and other Western-type diseases such as arteriosclerosis and diabetes. By increasing the amount of fibre or roughage in our diet they are hoping we will help reduce the incidence of such simple ailments as haemorrhoids, constipation, even varicose veins and also the more serious diseases like diverticular disease, cancer of the colon, appendicitis, gall stones and diabetes.

Most fibre found in foods is insoluble. It is not absorbed by the body but as it passes through the digestive tract it absorbs moisture increasing the volume and softness of the food thus speeding up its passage through the intestines.

Another function of dietary fibre is to slow down the absorption of sugar into the blood stream which gives a steadier blood sugar level, which is particularly important for diabetics. It is thought also that a certain type of fibre, particularly that found in high fibre vegetables (beans) and cereals, particularly oats is soluble and helps to control the cholesterol level of the blood which in turn may help to reduce the likelihood of arteriosclerosis.

The average person in the Western world has a daily fibre intake of about 20 g and it is thought that we should increase this to at least 30 to 35 g a day.

When the importance of fibre was first realized it was suggested that we simply increased our intake by sprinkling foods with high fibre bran. However, bran has a rather unusual taste and it takes someone of a very strong constitution to eat it in large quantities.

There are many ways of increasing daily fibre intake. You certainly don't have to become a health fanatic. Simply be a little more selective in your shopping and menu planning. Start serving meals that are based on the low cost, high protein, high fibre dried beans and peas rather than expensive meat, fish or chicken.

Don't be put off by the fact that you have to soak them overnight then cook them slowly. Most peas and beans are available in cans and these require no further cooking. They can simply be drained and served cold in salads, reheated and served as a vegetable, or added to numerous soups, stews and casseroles. Even the humble baked bean is an excellent source of fibre, 100 g/4 oz contains 7.3 grams.

Serve more fresh fruit and vegetables. Retain the peel or skins wherever possible. Scrub root vegetables rather than peeling them – you are less likely to loose the valuable minerals and vitamins that are situated just below the peel.

Vegetables that look stringy and fibrous are not necessarily those with the highest fibre content. Celery, despite its texture, has just under 2 grams of fibre per 100 g/4 oz whereas spinach which reduces to almost nothing when cooked, has 6 grams per 100 g/4 oz. Other vegetables high in fibre are broccoli, peas, sweetcorn (kernel corn), celeriac, leeks and potatoes baked in their jackets.

Create desserts based on fruit. Use puréed fruit instead of cream. Opt for high fibre fruit, such as dried fruits, dates, the currants, raspberries, damsons and passion fruit.

Buy high fibre breakfast cereals and use them in both sweet and savoury recipes. Serve wholewheat bread and use wholewheat flour for cooking. Experiment with your baking; substitute half the white flour in cake and biscuit recipes with wholewheat flour. It absorbs more liquid than white so you will have to add a little extra liquid.

Fortunately high fibre cooking is in keeping with the medical view that you should reduce the amount of animal protein, fats and sugar that you eat; and that you should obtain more protein from low fat, low sugar, plant sources.

High fibre eating is healthy eating – it is also low in cost. The recipes in this book show how easy it is to increase the fibre content of your meals both appetizingly and simply without spending a fortune on health foods.

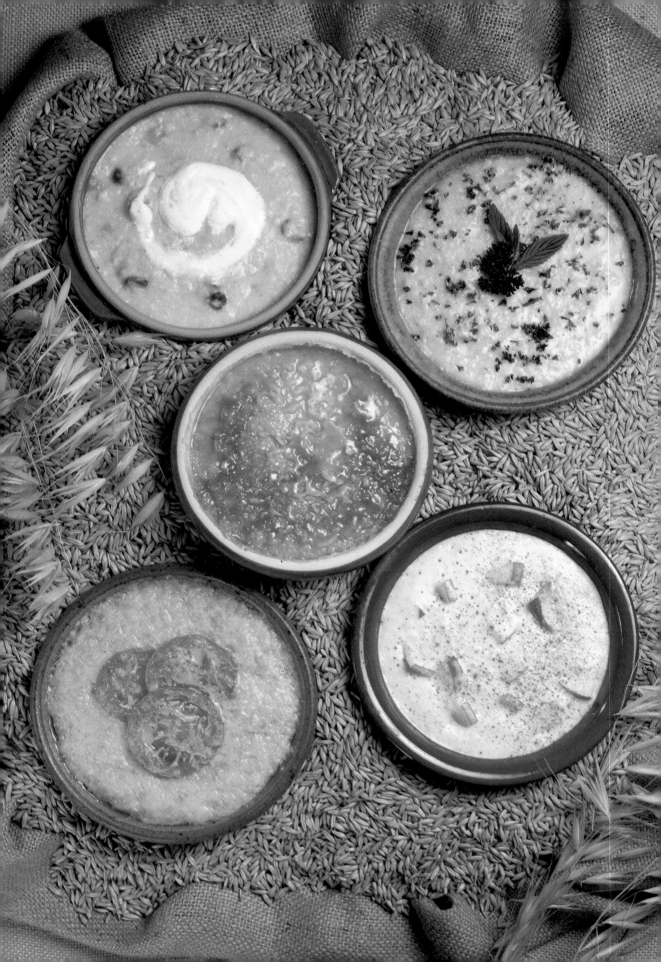

Breakfast & Brunch Dishes

METRIC/IMPERIAL	AMERICAN
100 g/4 oz butter	$\frac{1}{2}$ cup butter
50 g/2 oz sugar	$\frac{1}{4}$ cup sugar
100 g/4 oz strawberry or apricot jam	$\frac{1}{3}$ cup strawberry or apricot jam
100 g/4 oz rolled oats	$1\frac{1}{3}$ cup rolled oats
100 g/4 oz chopped nuts	1 cup chopped nuts
150 g/6 oz raisins or chopped dates	1 cup raisins or chopped dates

Combine the butter, sugar and jam in a large saucepan and cook over low heat, stirring constantly, until the mixture is well blended and smooth. Remove from the heat and stir in the oats and nuts. Mix until well coated then transfer the mixture to an ungreased 30 × 25 cm (12 × 10 inch) baking sheet. Bake in a preheated slow oven (170°C/325°F, Gas Mark 3) for 35 to 40 minutes or until golden. Stir occasionally. Remove from the oven, add the raisins and mix well. Transfer to an ungreased baking sheet to cool. Store in a tightly covered container.
Makes 600 g/1$\frac{1}{2}$ lb (4$\frac{1}{2}$ cups)

Porridge Variations

Rolled oats are high in fibre, especially the soluble variety, and they are also high in protein so a bowl of piping hot porridge served with milk makes a nutritious alternative to high-bran breakfast cereals. And porridge is surprisingly versatile . . .

Muesli Porridge Make porridge in usual way; add some dried fruit – sultanas, raisins, currants, soaked apricots or prunes – with chopped nuts or desiccated coconut. Top with a swirl of cream.

Fruit Porridge Make the porridge in the usual way and when thickened stir in an equal amount of sweetened apple purée (apple-sauce), adding a little ground cinnamon or nutmeg, diced apple and honey to taste.

Caramelized Porridge Make porridge in the usual way and sweeten to taste. Transfer to individual flameproof dishes and top each with a ring of pineapple. Sprinkle generously with brown sugar and place under a preheated grill (broiler) until sugar has melted.

Orange Porridge Make porridge using half orange juice and half water. Spoon into individual dishes and serve topped with fresh orange segments and cream.

Herby Porridge Make porridge in the usual way and add salt, freshly ground pepper and chopped fresh herbs to taste.

Porridge Mornay Cook porridge in the usual way. Allow 50–75 g/2–3 oz ($\frac{1}{2}$ cup) grated cheese per portion. Mix most of the cheese into the hot porridge and spoon into ovenproof dishes. Top with remaining cheese and brown under a preheated grill (broiler).

Rolled Oat Soufflé Make the porridge in the usual way using all milk. To each portion allow 2 eggs. Separate the yolks from the whites and stir into the hot porridge. Whisk the whites until stiff and fold into the porridge. Add sugar or honey to taste and spoon the mixture into individual soufflé dishes. Bake in a preheated moderately hot oven (190°C/375°F, Gas Mark 5) for about 20 minutes. Serve immediately.

Clockwise from top left: Muesli Porridge, Herby Porridge, Fruit Porridge, Porridge Mornay and Caramelized Porridge
(Photograph: Quaker Oats Ltd)

Kedgeree

METRIC/IMPERIAL	AMERICAN
175 g/6 oz brown rice	¾ cup brown rice
450 g/1 lb smoked haddock	1 lb smoked haddock
50 g/2 oz butter	¼ cup butter
2 hard-boiled eggs, chopped	2 hard-cooked eggs, chopped
2 teaspoons lemon juice	2 teaspoons lemon juice
salt	salt
freshly ground pepper	freshly ground pepper
1 tablespoon chopped parsley	1 tablespoon chopped parsley

Cook the rice in boiling salted water according to packet instructions, about 40 minutes. Drain when tender and keep hot. Remove the skin from the smoked fish and dice. Melt the butter in a large saucepan and gently sauté the fish for 5 minutes. Stir in the cooked rice, chopped eggs and lemon juice. Heat through. Adjust seasoning to taste and serve sprinkled with parsley.
Serves 4

Orange and Prune Crunch

METRIC/IMPERIAL	AMERICAN
175 ml/6 fl oz plain yogurt	¾ cup plain yogurt
¼ teaspoon ground ginger	¼ teaspoon ground ginger
2 large oranges	2 large oranges
75 g/3 oz cooked prunes, chopped	½ cup chopped cooked prunes
50 g/2 oz muesli-type breakfast cereal or rolled oats	½ cup Granola breakfast cereal or rolled oats
honey to serve	honey to serve

Combine the yogurt and the ginger. Remove the skin, pith and membrane from the oranges and slice finely. Mix with the yogurt, chopped prunes and breakfast cereal. Spoon into individual dishes and serve accompanied with honey to sweeten.
Serves 4

Sausage Bran Burgers

METRIC/IMPERIAL	AMERICAN
1 egg, beaten	1 egg, beaten
4 tablespoons milk	4 tablespoons milk
50 g/2 oz All Bran breakfast cereal	1 cup All Bran breakfast cereal
450 g/1 lb pork or beef sausage meat	1 lb pork or beef sausage mince
salt	salt
freshly ground pepper	freshly ground pepper

Mix together the egg, milk and bran cereal and allow to stand until the milk has been absorbed. Mix this with the sausage meat and seasoning. Divide the mixture into 8 and shape into burgers. At this stage the burgers may be covered and refrigerated overnight. Place the burgers on a baking sheet and bake in a hot oven (200°C/400°F, Gas Mark 6) for about 30 minutes or until cooked through. Serve with baked beans in tomato sauce or grilled tomatoes.
Serves 4

Oven-baked Tomato Toasts

METRIC/IMPERIAL	AMERICAN
5 eggs	5 eggs
3 tablespoons milk	3 tablespoons milk
few drops Worcestershire sauce	few drops Worcestershire sauce
salt	salt
freshly ground pepper	freshly ground pepper
50 oz/2 oz Bran Flakes breakfast cereal, crushed	2 cups crushed Bran Flakes breakfast cereal
4 slices wholewheat bread	4 slices wholewheat bread
4 small tomatoes, sliced	4 small tomatoes, sliced

Beat one egg with the milk, Worcestershire sauce, salt and pepper. Place the crushed Bran Flakes on a plate. Remove the crusts from the bread and cut each slice in two. Dip the bread into the egg mixture and then in to the crumbs, coating evenly. Place the bread in an ovenproof serving dish and arrange the tomato slices on top. Bake in a moderately hot oven (190°C/375°F, Gas Mark 5) for 15 minutes. While bread is baking fry the eggs in a little oil. Top each slice with a fried egg and serve immediately.
Serves 4

Herring and Oatmeal Fries

METRIC/IMPERIAL	AMERICAN
1 kg/2 lb fresh herring	2 lb fresh herring
flour for dusting	flour for dusting
100 g/4 oz rolled oats	1⅓ cup rolled oats
salt	salt
freshly ground pepper	freshly ground pepper
1 teaspoon dry mustard	1 teaspoon dry mustard
2 eggs, beaten	2 eggs, beaten
oil for deep frying	oil for deep frying
2 oranges, sliced	2 oranges, sliced
parsley to garnish	parsley to garnish

Clean and remove the heads from the herrings. Split along the stomach, open the fish and place, skin side uppermost, on a board. Press firmly along the back of the fish to loosen the back bone. Turn the fish over and remove the back bone. Wash and dry the fish then cut into 5 cm (2 inch) strips and dust thoroughly with flour. Mix the oats with seasoning and mustard. Dip the fish strips in egg then coat with the rolled oats. Heat oil to 180°C/350°F. Add the fish in batches and deep fry until golden, about 5 minutes. Dry well on absorbent kitchen paper and keep warm while frying the rest of the fish. Arrange the orange slices on a plate, pile on the fried fish strips and serve piping hot, garnished with parsley.
Serves 4 to 6

Crunchy Fruit Compote

METRIC/IMPERIAL	AMERICAN
250 g/8 oz mixed dried fruit (apricots, peaches, prunes etc)	1¼ cups mixed dried fruit (apricots, peaches, prunes etc)
150 ml/¼ pint water	⅔ cup water
1 tablespoon honey	1 tablespoon honey
juice of ½ lemon	juice of ½ lemon
45 g/1½ oz butter	3 tablespoons butter
2 tablespoons demerara sugar	2 tablespoons brown sugar
75 g/3 oz muesli-type breakfast cereal	1 cup Swiss muesli-type breakfast cereal

Place the dried fruits in a bowl with enough water to cover and leave to soak overnight. The next day, drain the fruit well then place in a saucepan with the 150 ml/¼ pint (⅔ cup) water, honey and lemon juice. Bring to the boil, cover and cook gently until the fruits are tender, about 20 minutes. Transfer to an ovenproof dish. Melt the butter in a small saucepan and stir in the sugar and breakfast cereal. Sprinkle this mixture over the fruit and place under a preheated hot grill (broiler) until golden. Serve warm with plain yogurt.
Serves 2

Breakfast Bacon Squares

METRIC/IMPERIAL	AMERICAN
175 g/6 oz butter or margarine	¾ cup butter or margarine
150 g/5 oz sugar	⅔ cup sugar
1 egg	1 egg
1 teaspoon vanilla essence	1 teaspoon vanilla
100 g/4 oz plain flour	1 cup all-purpose flour
½ teaspoon bicarbonate of soda	½ teaspoon baking soda
100 g/4 oz rolled oats	1⅓ cups rolled oats
100 g/4 oz Cheddar cheese, grated	1 cup shredded Cheddar cheese
50 g/2 oz wheatgerm or finely chopped nuts	½ cup wheatgerm or finely chopped nuts
6 rashers bacon, fried until crisp	6 slices bacon, fried until crisp

Beat together the butter, sugar, egg and vanilla until the mixture is well blended. Sift together the flour and soda and fold in to the butter mixture with the oats, cheese, wheatgerm or nuts and crumbled bacon. Drop tablespoonfuls of the mixture on to greased baking sheets and bake in a preheated moderate oven (180°C/350°F, Gas Mark 4) for 12 to 15 minutes or until the edges are golden. Cool for 1 minute then transfer to a wire cooling rack.
Makes about 25

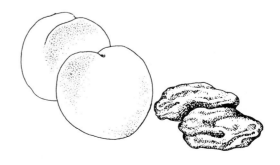

Poached Eggs on Bran Cakes

METRIC/IMPERIAL	AMERICAN
1 egg, beaten	1 egg, beaten
150 ml/¼ pint milk	⅔ cup milk
75 g/3 oz All Bran breakfast cereal	1½ cups All Bran breakfast cereal
25 g/1 oz plain flour	¼ cup all-purpose flour
salt	salt
freshly ground pepper	freshly ground pepper
4 eggs	4 eggs
a little butter	a little butter

Mix together the beaten egg, milk and All Bran breakfast cereal. Allow to stand for about 10 minutes or until all the liquid has been absorbed. Stir in the flour, salt and pepper. Divide the mixture into 4 and place on a greased baking sheet. Spread into four 10 cm/4 inch squares and bake in a hot oven (200°C/400°F, Gas Mark 6) for about 20 minutes or until crisp. Meanwhile poach the eggs. Spread the hot bran cakes with a little butter and top each with a poached egg. Serve with grilled bacon, tomatoes and mushrooms.
Serves 4

Yogurt and Oat Muesli

METRIC/IMPERIAL	AMERICAN
250 ml plain yogurt	1 cup plain yogurt
75 g/3 oz rolled oats	1 cup rolled oats
4 tablespoons raisins	4 tablespoons raisins
3 tablespoons sugar	3 tablespoons sugar
2 eating apples, grated	2 apples, shredded
4 tablespoons chopped walnuts	4 tablespoons chopped walnuts
juice of 1 lemon	juice of 1 lemon

Put the yogurt into a large mixing bowl and add all the remaining ingredients. Mix thoroughly and leave to stand for a few hours, or refrigerate overnight before serving.
Serves 2

Store-cupboard Muesli

METRIC/IMPERIAL	AMERICAN
225 g/8 oz rolled oats	2⅔ cup rolled oats
100 g/4 oz Bran Flakes breakfast cereal	1 cup Bran Flakes breakfast cereal
50 g/2 oz chopped nuts	½ cup chopped nuts
50 g/2 oz seedless raisins and coarsely chopped dried fruit	⅓ cup seedless raisins and coarsely chopped dried fruit

Place the rolled oats in a sieve and shake vigorously to remove the "flour". Place the oats in a mixing bowl and mix in all the other ingredients. Store in an airtight container and serve at breakfast with a little chopped fresh fruit and some plain yogurt.
Makes about 450 g/1 lb

Lemon Breakfast Muffins

METRIC/IMPERIAL	AMERICAN
50 g/2 oz All Bran breakfast cereal	1 cup All Bran breakfast cereal
150 ml/¼ pint milk	⅔ cup milk
50 g/2 oz butter	¼ cup butter
50 g/2 oz sugar	4 tablespoons sugar
1 egg, beaten	1 egg, beaten
2 tablespoons chopped walnuts	2 tablespoons chopped walnuts
3 tablespoons lemon curd	3 tablespoons lemon curd
100 g/4 oz plain flour	1 cup all-purpose flour
3 teaspoons baking powder	3 teaspoons baking powder

Place the breakfast cereal in a bowl with the milk and leave until soft. Add the butter, sugar, egg, nuts and lemon curd and beat until the mixture is smooth. Sift together the flour and baking powder and gently fold into the milk mixture. Do not overmix. Spoon mixture into 15 greased deep bun tins (muffin pans) and bake in a hot oven (200°C/400°F, Gas Mark 6) for 20–25 minutes or until golden and springy to touch. Serve warm with butter.
Makes 15
Note:
For a higher fibre content use wholewheat flour but increase the amount of milk used by 2 tablespoons.

Store-cupboard Muesli

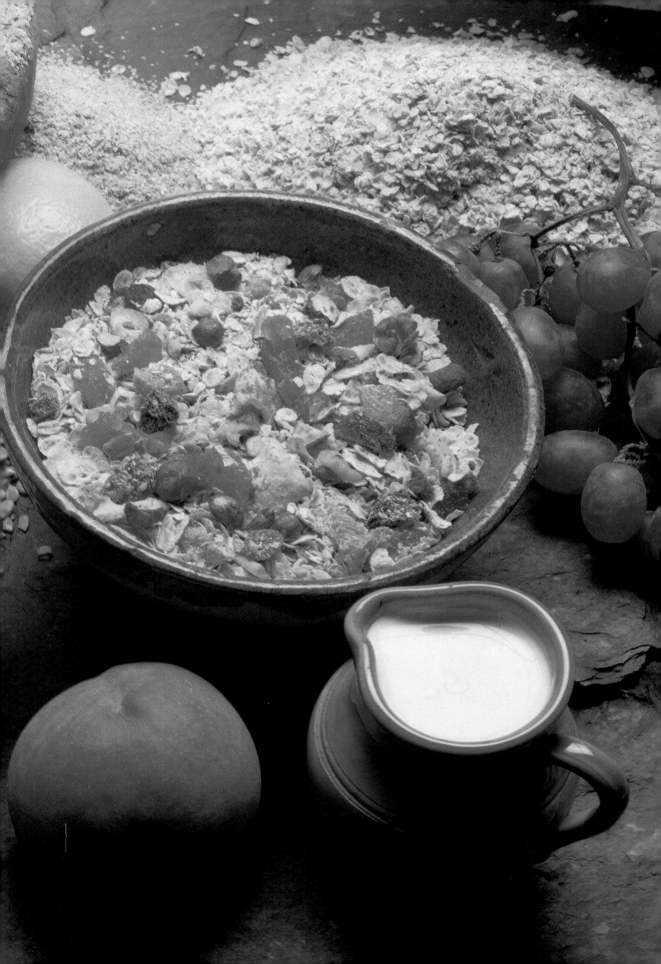

Bean Brunch

METRIC/IMPERIAL	AMERICAN
2 tablespoons oil	2 tablespoons oil
1 large onion, sliced	1 large onion, sliced
450 g/1 lb potatoes, cooked and diced	2 cups cooked and diced potatoes
2 × 225 g/8 oz can curried baked beans in tomato sauce	2 × 8 oz can curried baked beans in tomato sauce
salt	salt
freshly ground pepper	freshly ground pepper
4 eggs	4 eggs
50 g/2 oz Cheddar cheese, grated	$\frac{1}{2}$ cup shredded Cheddar cheese

Heat the oil in a saucepan and sauté the onion slices until transparent. Stir in the cooked potatoes, beans and salt and pepper to taste. Transfer the mixture to an ovenproof serving dish. Make 4 hollows in the mixture and break an egg into each one. Sprinkle with the cheese and bake in a hot oven (200°C/400°F, Gas Mark 6) for 15 to 20 minutes or until the eggs are cooked and the beans heated through. Serve immediately.
Serves 4

Bean and Squeak

METRIC/IMPERIAL	AMERICAN
450 g/1 lb potatoes, boiled and mashed	1 lb potatoes, boiled and mashed
450 g/1 lb cabbage, shredded and cooked	1 lb cabbage, shredded and cooked
1 × 284 g/10 oz can haricot beans, drained	1 × 10 oz can navy beans, drained
salt	salt
freshly ground pepper	freshly ground pepper
50 g/2 oz butter	$\frac{1}{4}$ cup butter
4 spring onions, finely chopped	4 scallions, finely chopped
2 tablespoons oil	2 tablespoons oil

Mix together the potatoes, cabbage and drained beans. Beat in the salt, pepper and butter. Stir in the spring onions (scallions). Heat the oil in a large frying pan (skillet) and turn the mixture into it. Cook until the base is golden. Serve with fried or poached eggs.
Serves 4

Lentil Patties

METRIC/IMPERIAL	AMERICAN
2 tablespoons oil	2 tablespoons oil
1 clove garlic, peeled and crushed	1 clove garlic, peeled and crushed
1 onion, finely chopped	1 onion, finely chopped
1 celery stick, chopped	1 celery stalk, chopped
1 carrot, chopped	1 carrot, chopped
225 g/8 oz brown lentils	1 cup brown lentils
450 ml/$\frac{3}{4}$ pint water	2 cups water
salt	salt
freshly ground pepper	freshly ground pepper
4 tablespoons wholewheat flour	4 tablespoons wholewheat flour
$\frac{1}{2}$ teaspoon ground ginger	$\frac{1}{2}$ teaspoon ground ginger
$\frac{1}{2}$ teaspoon ground cumin	$\frac{1}{2}$ teaspoon ground cumin
1 teaspoon curry powder	1 teaspoon curry powder
1 tablespoon mango chutney, chopped	1 tablespoon chopped mango chutney
oil for shallow frying	oil for shallow frying
Dressing:	**Dressing:**
150 ml/$\frac{1}{4}$ pint plain yogurt	$\frac{2}{3}$ cup plain yogurt
1 glove garlic, crushed	1 clove garlic, crushed
1 tablespoon chopped parsley	1 tablespoon chopped parsley

Heat the oil in a large pan. Add the garlic, onion, celery and carrot and sauté until the vegetables begin to soften. Add the lentils, water, salt and pepper. Bring to the boil, then lower the heat, cover and simmer for about 1 hour until the lentils are soft and all the liquid is absorbed. Add 2 tablespoons flour, the spices and chutney to the pan and mix well. Continue to cook gently for 2 to 3 minutes, stirring constantly. Adjust the seasoning, if necessary. Turn the mixture onto a plate and leave until cool enough to handle.

Divide the mixture into 18 equal pieces and form each one into a patty, about 1 cm/$\frac{1}{2}$ inch thick. Coat with the remaining flour. Heat a little oil in a frying pan (skillet) and fry the lentil patties, a few at a time, until crisp and golden brown, turning once.

For the dressing, mix together the yogurt, garlic and parsley. Serve the patties on a bed of rice, topped with the yogurt dressing.
Serves 6

Brown Rice Piperade

METRIC/IMPERIAL	AMERICAN
2 tablespoons oil	2 tablespoons oil
1 large onion, chopped	1 large onion, chopped
2 carrots, diced	2 carrots, diced
450 g/1 lb spinach, shredded	1 lb spinach, shredded
1 tablespoon chopped parsley	1 tablespoon chopped parsley
225 g/8 oz brown rice, cooked	1 cup cooked brown rice
salt	salt
freshly ground pepper	freshly ground pepper
3 eggs, beaten	3 eggs, beaten
½ teaspoon Worcestershire sauce	½ teaspoon Worcestershire sauce

Heat the oil in a large frying pan (skillet). Add the onion, carrots and spinach. Stir-fry until the onions are translucent and spinach tender. Add the parsley, rice, salt and pepper to the frying pan (skillet). Add the beaten eggs and the Worcestershire sauce. Stir the mixture until the eggs have set. Serve immediately.
Serves 4
Variation:
Add 4 tablespoons of toasted flaked (slivered) almonds.

Mornay Medley

METRIC/IMPERIAL	AMERICAN
1 × 284 g/10 oz can butter beans	1 × 10 oz can lima beans
1 × 284 g/10 oz can new potatoes	1 × 10 oz can new potatoes
3 eggs	3 eggs
175 ml/6 fl oz single cream	¾ cup light cream
50 g/2 oz Cheddar cheese, grated	½ cup shredded Cheddar cheese
1 teaspoon made mustard	1 teaspoon prepared mustard
salt	salt
freshly ground pepper	freshly ground pepper
pinch ground nutmeg or mace	pinch ground nutmeg or mace
chopped parsley to garnish	chopped parsley to garnish

Heat the beans and potatoes by standing the opened cans in a pan of boiling water. Add the eggs to the water and boil for 10 minutes. Lift out the cans with a cloth, drain the contents and place in an ovenproof dish. Shell and quarter the eggs and add to the vegetables. Place the cream in a small saucepan. Add the cheese, mustard, salt, pepper and nutmeg or mace. Bring to the boil, stirring all the time with a wooden spoon. Pour over the egg and vegetables and garnish with chopped parsley. Serve at once with a crisp salad or green vegetable.
Serves 4

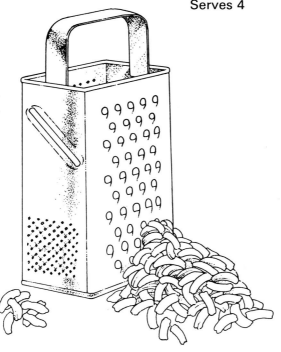

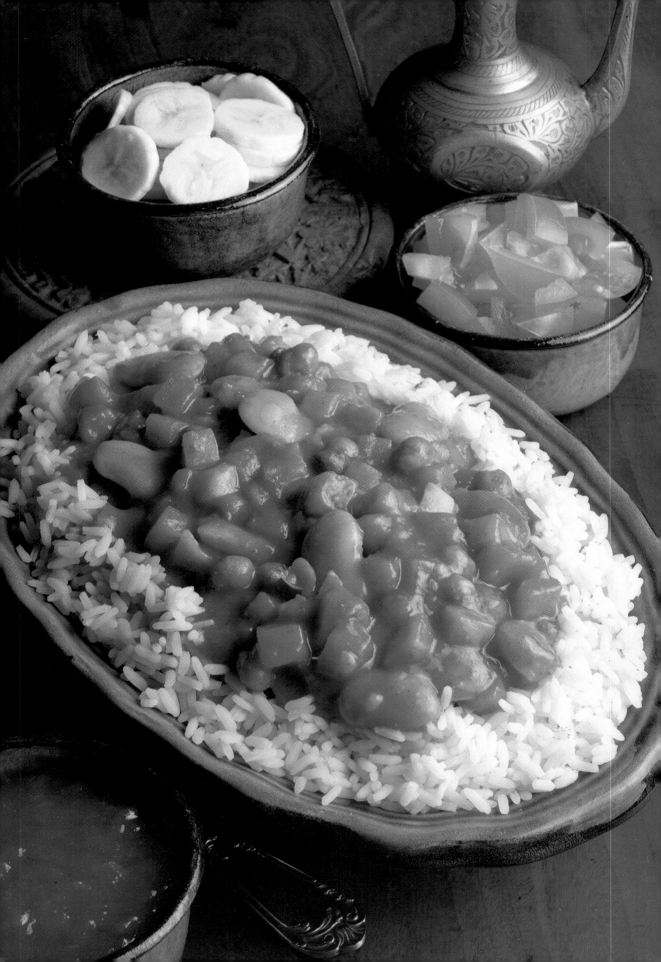

Vegetarian Dishes

Instant Vegetable Curry

METRIC/IMPERIAL	AMERICAN
2 tablespoons oil	2 tablespoons oil
1 onion, sliced	1 onion, sliced
2 teaspoons curry powder	2 teaspoons curry powder
1 tablespoon plain flour	1 tablespoon all-purpose flour
1 × 439 g/15½ oz can butter beans	1 × 16 oz can lima beans
1 × 425 g/15 oz can mulligatawny soup	1 × 16 oz can mulligatawny soup
1 × 538 g/1 lb 3 oz can mixed vegetables	1 × 19 oz can mixed vegetables

Heat the oil in a large saucepan, add the onion and curry powder and sauté until the onion has softened. Stir in the flour and cook for a few minutes then add the drained beans, soup and mixed vegetables with their liquor. Bring to the boil stirring continuously. Cook for about 5 minutes then serve with boiled brown rice.
Serves 4

Oatmeal Soup

METRIC/IMPERIAL	AMERICAN
40 g/1½ oz butter	3 tablespoons butter
2 onions, chopped	2 onions, chopped
2 carrots, diced	2 carrots, diced
1 small turnip, diced	1 small turnip, diced
2 leeks, sliced	2 leeks, sliced
100 g/4 oz red lentils	½ cup lentils
50 g/2 oz rolled oats	⅔ cup rolled oats
600 ml/1 pint homemade vegetable stock	2¾ cups homemade vegetable stock
salt	salt
freshly ground pepper	freshly ground pepper
1 tablespoon chopped parsley	1 tablespoon chopped parsley
600 ml/1 pint milk	2¾ cups milk

Heat the butter in a large saucepan. Add the prepared vegetables, cover the pan and allow the vegetables to cook gently for 5 minutes. Sprinkle over the lentils and oats, fry gently with the vegetables for about 2 minutes. Slowly add the stock and bring the mixture to the boil. Reduce heat and simmer gently for 30 minutes. Add the seasoning and parsley then gradually stir in the milk. Bring the soup back to the boil and serve.
Serves 6

Instant Vegetable Curry
(Photograph: Canned Food Advisory Service)

Italian Bean Soup

METRIC/IMPERIAL	AMERICAN
225 g/8 oz dried white beans (haricot, butter beans, etc)	1 cup dried white beans (navy, lima, etc)
600 ml/1 pint water	2½ cups water
1 large onion, chopped	1 large onion, chopped
1 clove garlic, crushed	1 clove garlic, crushed
1 celery stick, sliced	1 celery stalk, sliced
1 large carrot, sliced	1 large carrot, sliced
4 tomatoes, skinned and chopped	4 tomatoes, skinned and chopped
finely grated rind and juice of ½ lemon	finely grated rind and juice of ½ lemon
1 bay leaf	1 bay leaf
salt	salt
freshly ground pepper	freshly ground pepper
2 tablespoons chopped parsley (optional)	2 tablespoons chopped parsley (optional)

Put the beans in a large bowl, cover with the water, then leave to soak overnight. Alternatively, pour over boiling water and soak for several hours. Drain the beans, reserving the water. Make up to 1.2 litres/2 pints/5 cups with stock or more water. Place the beans and liquid in a large pan, then add all the remaining ingredients, except the parsley. Bring to the boil, then lower the heat, cover and simmer for 1 to 1½ hours until the beans are tender, adding more water if necessary. Discard the bay leaf.

Transfer about half the beans and some of the liquid into an electric blender. Work to a smooth purée. Return the purée to the soup and bring to the boil, stirring constantly. Taste and adjust the seasoning, and add more liquid if the soup is too thick. Sprinkle with parsley if liked, and serve hot.
Serves 4 to 6

Mediterranean Lentil Stew

METRIC/IMPERIAL	AMERICAN
2 tablespoons oil	2 tablespoons oil
2 onions, peeled and chopped	2 onions, peeled and chopped
1 clove garlic, crushed	1 clove garlic, crushed
2 celery sticks, sliced	2 celery sticks, sliced
4 small courgettes, sliced	4 small zucchini, sliced
4 tomatoes, skinned and quartered	4 tomatoes, skinned and quartered
900 ml/1½ pints water or stock	3¾ cups water or stock
¼ teaspoon ground coriander	¼ teaspoon ground coriander
salt	salt
freshly ground pepper	freshly ground pepper
225 g/8 oz brown lentils	1 cup brown lentils
2 tablespoons chopped parsley (optional)	2 tablespoons chopped parsley (optional)

Heat the oil in a large pan. Add the onions, garlic, celery and courgettes (zucchini) and fry gently for 10 minutes until lightly browned, stirring frequently. Add the tomatoes, water or stock, coriander and salt and pepper to taste. Bring to the boil. Add the lentils, then cover and simmer for 1 to 1½ hours until the lentils are tender.

Alternatively, transfer the ingredients to a casserole, cover and bake in a preheated moderate oven (180°C/350°F, Gas Mark 4) for 1½ to 2 hours. Sprinkle with the chopped parsley, if liked, and serve hot.
Serves 4

Brown Rice Ratatouille

METRIC/IMPERIAL	AMERICAN
4 tablespoons cooking oil	4 tablespoons cooking oil
1 green pepper, cored, seeded and chopped	1 green pepper, cored, seeded and chopped
225 g/8 oz courgettes, sliced	2 cups zucchini, sliced
2 small aubergines, sliced	2 small eggplants, sliced
1 onion, sliced	1 onion, sliced
100 g/4 oz brown rice	$\frac{1}{2}$ cup brown rice
1 × 397 g/14 oz can tomatoes	1 × 16 oz can tomatoes
250 ml stock	1 cup stock
salt	salt
freshly ground pepper	freshly ground pepper
1 clove garlic, crushed	1 clove garlic, crushed
grated cheese to serve	shredded cheese to serve

Heat the oil in a saucepan and lightly sauté the pepper, courgettes (zucchini), aubergine (egg-plant), onion and brown rice. When mixture is well coated with oil and beginning to turn golden add the canned tomatoes with their juice, the stock, seasoning and garlic. Bring to the boil, reduce the heat, cover and simmer gently until the brown rice is cooked, about 40 minutes. Stir occasionally, adding more hot stock if the mixture looks as though it is drying up. Serve hot, passing around a bowl of grated (shredded) cheese separately.
Serves 2 to 4

Cheese and Bean Mousse

METRIC/IMPERIAL	AMERICAN
1 × 439 g/15$\frac{1}{2}$ oz can baked beans	1 × 16 oz can baked beans
125 g/5 oz cottage cheese	$\frac{1}{2}$ cup cottage cheese
1 teaspoon dried mint	1 teaspoon dried mint
salt	salt
freshly ground pepper	freshly ground pepper
1 tablespoon lemon juice	1 tablespoon lemon juice
15 g/$\frac{1}{2}$ oz powdered gelatine	1 envelope unflavored gelatin
2 tablespoons water	2 tablespoons water

Tip the beans into the goblet of a blender or food processor with the cottage cheese, mint,

salt, pepper and lemon juice. Blend until smooth. Dissolve the gelatine slowly in the water in a bowl over a pan of hot water. Add to the mixture and stir well. Pour into a 750 ml/1$\frac{1}{4}$ pint (3 cup) wetted dish, chill until set, turn out and serve with salad.
Serves 4

Bean and Herb Soufflé

METRIC/IMPERIAL	AMERICAN
100 g/4 oz butter beans	$\frac{1}{2}$ cup lima beans
600 ml/1 pint water	2$\frac{1}{2}$ cups water
150 ml/$\frac{1}{4}$ pint milk	$\frac{2}{3}$ cup milk
1 large onion, grated	1 large onion, grated
4 tomatoes, skinned and chopped	4 tomatoes, skinned and chopped
1 tablespoon chopped parsley	1 tablespoon chopped parsley
1 tablespoon chopped thyme	1 tablespoon chopped thyme
1 teaspoon chopped sage	1 teaspoon chopped sage
salt	salt
freshly ground pepper	freshly ground pepper
4 eggs, separated	4 eggs, separated

Put the beans in a large bowl, cover with the water, then leave to soak overnight. Alternatively, pour over boiling water and soak for several hours.

Transfer the beans and water to a pan, then bring to the boil. Lower the heat, cover and simmer for about 1$\frac{1}{2}$ hours until the beans are soft, adding more water if necessary. Drain the beans, return to the rinsed-out pan and mash well. Add the milk and onion and bring to the boil, stirring constantly. Simmer for 1 minute. Remove the pan from the heat, then stir in the tomatoes, herbs and salt and pepper to taste. Stir in the egg yolks and leave to cool slightly.

Beat the egg whites until just stiff, then fold into the bean sauce. Pour the mixture into a 1.5 litre/2$\frac{1}{2}$ pint/6$\frac{1}{4}$ cup soufflé dish. Bake in a preheated moderate oven (180°C/350°F, Gas Mark 4) for 1 hour until the soufflé has risen and is lightly browned on top. Serve immediately.
Serves 4 to 6

Bean and Peanut Loaf

METRIC/IMPERIAL	AMERICAN
1 × 225 g/8 oz packet sage and onion stuffing mix	1 × ½ lb package sage and onion forcemeat mix
250 ml/8 fl oz boiling water	1 cup boiling water
1 × 450 g/16 oz can baked beans	1 × 16 oz can baked beans
salt	salt
freshly ground pepper	freshly ground pepper
1 egg, beaten	1 egg, beaten
2 tablespoons single cream	2 tablespoons light cream
75 g/3 oz peanuts, chopped	½ cup chopped peanuts
Topping:	**Topping:**
1 tomato, sliced	1 tomato, sliced
parsley sprigs	parsley sprigs

Grease and line the bottom of a 1 kg/2 lb loaf pan. Mix the stuffing mix with the boiling water then stir in the baked beans, salt, pepper, egg, cream and nuts. Spoon the mixture into the prepared loaf tin and level the top. Cover with greased foil and bake in a preheated moderate oven (190°C/375°F, Gas Mark 5) for 45 minutes. Carefully turn out the loaf on to a serving dish and serve hot or cold topped with tomato slices and parsley.
Serves 6
Variation:
Add 100 g/4 oz (1 cup) grated Cheddar cheese if liked.

Bean and Cheese Pancakes

METRIC/IMPERIAL	AMERICAN
100 g/4 oz wholewheat flour	1 cup wholewheat flour
1 egg	1 egg
150 ml/¼ pint water	⅔ cup water
150 ml/¼ pint milk	⅔ cup milk
1 teaspoon dried dill	1 teaspoon dried dill
oil for frying	oil for frying
Filling:	**Filling:**
225 g/8 oz cottage cheese	1 cup cottage cheese
salt	salt
freshly ground pepper	freshly ground pepper
2 × 225 g/8 oz cans curried beans with sultanas	2 × 8 oz cans curried beans with golden raisins
Topping:	**Topping:**
150 ml/¼ pint soured cream	⅔ cup sour cream
chopped chives	chopped chives

For the batter, place the flour in a mixing bowl, make a well in the centre, add the egg and half the water and beat to form a smooth paste. Gradually whisk in the milk and enough of the remaining water to give a batter the consistency of thick cream. Add the dill and seasoning to taste. Lightly oil a small pancake pan, about 15 cm (6 inches) across. Add a spoonful of batter to the pan, tilt the pan to coat evenly then cook lightly over a medium heat until golden on the underside. Turn the pancake and brown on the other side. Transfer the pancake to a plate and continue making pancakes until all the batter has been used. For the filling, mix the cottage cheese with the salt, pepper, and the curried beans. Divide the filling between the pancakes and roll up each one. Arrange on a greased ovenproof serving dish, cover with foil and cook in a moderately hot oven (190°C/375°F, Gas Mark 5) for about 8 minutes. Meanwhile heat the sour cream over a low heat, spoon over the heated pancakes and serve sprinkled with chopped chives.
Serves 4 to 6

Bean and Peanut Loaf; Bean and Cheese Pancakes (Photograph: Heinz Baked Beans)

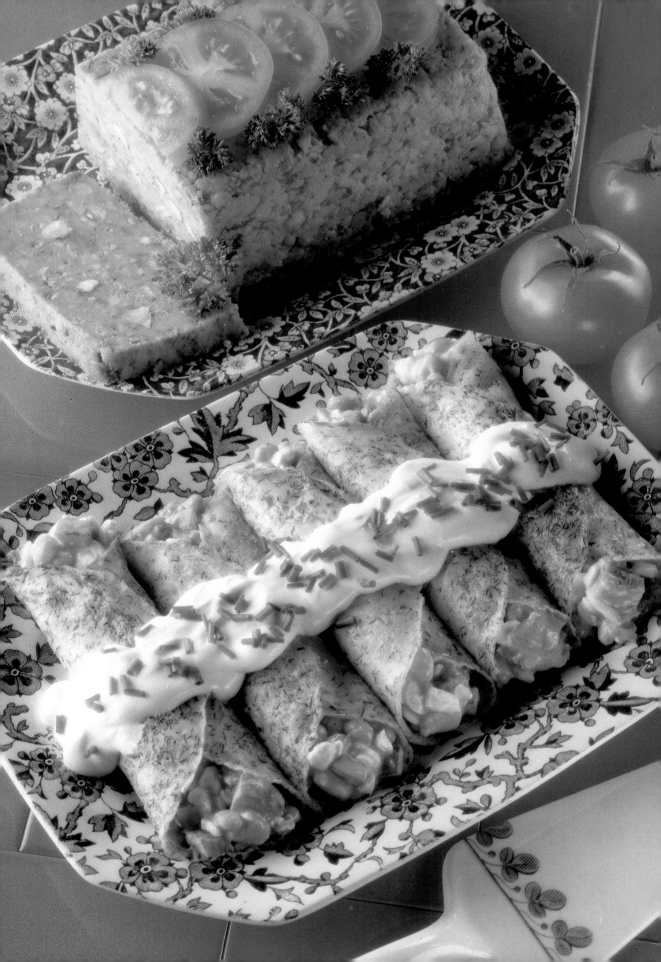

Broccoli and Nut Squares

METRIC/IMPERIAL	AMERICAN
2 × 10 oz packets frozen broccoli	2 × 10 oz packages frozen broccoli
100 g/4 oz plain flour	1 cup all-purpose flour
1 teaspoon baking powder	1 teaspoon baking powder
salt	salt
freshly ground pepper	freshly ground pepper
$\frac{1}{4}$ teaspoon ground nutmeg	$\frac{1}{4}$ teaspoon ground nutmeg
3 eggs, beaten	3 eggs, beaten
250 g/8 oz Cheddar cheese, grated	2 cups shredded Cheddar cheese
4 tablespoons flaked almonds	4 tablespoons slivered almonds

Cook broccoli according to packet (package) instructions. Drain well and transfer to a blender or food processor. Purée until smooth. Alternatively finely chop the broccoli. Sift the flour and baking powder into a mixing bowl. Add salt, pepper, nutmeg and the eggs. Stir to combine then stir in the broccoli, cheese and almonds. Transfer the mixture to a well greased 30 × 20 cm/12 × 8 inch baking dish. Bake in a preheated moderate oven (180°C/350°F, Gas Mark 4) for 30 to 40 minutes or until set. Serve warm, cut into squares.
Serves 6

Baked Bean Hummus

METRIC/IMPERIAL	AMERICAN
1 × 450 g/16 oz can baked beans	1 × 16 oz can baked beans
3 cloves garlic, crushed	3 cloves garlic, crushed
4 tablespoons olive oil	4 tablespoons olive oil
2 slices wholewheat bread, crusts removed	2 slices wholewheat bread, crusts removed
salt	salt
freshly ground pepper	freshly ground pepper
lemon juice to taste	lemon juice to taste
To serve:	**To serve:**
pitta bread	pitta bread
black and green olives	black and green olives

Place the canned beans into a blender or food processor with the garlic and olive oil. Add the bread to the blender with the salt, pepper and lemon juice. Blend until mixture is smooth and creamy, adding more olive oil or bread if necessary to adjust the consistency of the hummus. Stir in seasoning and lemon juice to taste. Serve with pitta bread and olives.
Serves 6 to 8

Savoury Bean Cheesecake

METRIC/IMPERIAL	AMERICAN
Base:	**Base:**
100 g/4 oz water biscuits	1$\frac{1}{2}$ cups cracker crumbs
1 tablespoon black poppy seeds	1 tablespoon black poppy seeds
50 g/2 oz butter, melted	4 tablespoons melted butter
Filling:	**Filling:**
225 g/8 oz cream cheese	1 cup cream cheese
300 ml/$\frac{1}{2}$ pint soured cream	1$\frac{1}{4}$ cups sour cream
2 eggs	2 eggs
1 × 450 g/16 oz can baked beans	1 × 16 oz can baked beans
salt	salt
freshly ground pepper	freshly ground pepper
1 clove garlic, crushed	1 clove garlic, crushed
2 tablespoons powdered gelatine	2 envelopes unflavored gelatin
3 tablespoons very hot water	3 tablespoons very hot water
To garnish:	**To garnish:**
sliced cucumber	sliced cucumber
paprika	paprika

For the base, mix the crushed biscuits (cracker crumbs) with the poppy seeds and melted butter. Press the mixture evenly over the base of a greased 20 cm (8 inch) loose-bottomed (spring-form) cake pan. Chill for 30 minutes. For the filling, place the cream cheese, soured cream, eggs, baked beans, salt, pepper and garlic into a blender or food processor and blend until smooth. Dissolve the gelatine in the very hot water. Add to the cheese mixture and mix well. Pour into the prepared tin. Refrigerate the cheesecake until the filling has set. To serve, remove from the pan and decorate with cucumber slices and paprika.
Serves 6 to 8

Vegetarian Wholewheat Pasta

METRIC/IMPERIAL	AMERICAN
350–500 g/¾–1 lb wholewheat noodles	3–4 cups wholewheat noodles
4 tablespoons oil	4 tablespoons oil
2 large onions, sliced	2 large onions, sliced
450 g/1 lb courgettes, sliced	1 lb zucchini, sliced
3 peppers – preferably 1 green, 1 red and 1 yellow, cored, seeded and chopped	3 peppers – preferably 1 green, 1 red and 1 yellow, cored, seeded and chopped
1 × 425 g/15 oz can tomatoes	1 × 16 oz can tomatoes
½ teaspoon dried basil or oregano	½ teaspoon dried basil or oregano
salt	salt
freshly ground pepper	freshly ground pepper
pinch of sugar	pinch of sugar
100 g/4 oz Cheddar cheese, grated	1 cup shredded Cheddar cheese

Cook the noodles in plenty of boiling salted water until just tender. Meanwhile, heat the oil in a saucepan and sauté the onion for two minutes. Add the courgettes (zucchini) and peppers and sauté for a further two minutes, stirring. Add the tomatoes, basil or oregano, salt, pepper and sugar and cook gently until the vegetables are tender. Drain the noodles well and transfer to a heated serving dish. Pile the sauce on top and serve immediately. Pass the cheese around separately.
Serves 4

Vegetarian Medley

METRIC/IMPERIAL	AMERICAN
40 g/1½ oz butter	3 tablespoons butter
½ teaspoon cumin seed	½ teaspoon cumin seed
1 teaspoon ground coriander	1 teaspoon ground coriander
½ teaspoon ground ginger	½ teaspoon ground ginger
¼ teaspoon cayenne pepper	¼ teaspoon cayenne pepper
salt	salt
2 × 439 g/15½ oz cans peas	2 × 16 oz cans peas
100 g/4 oz ground cashew nuts	1 cup ground cashew nuts
1 × 425 g/15 oz can new potatoes	1 × 16 oz can new potatoes
4 tomatoes sliced	4 tomatoes, sliced
25 g/1 oz butter, melted	2 tablespoons melted butter

Melt the 40 g/1½ oz (3 tablespoons) of butter in a saucepan, add the cumin seed and cook for a few seconds. Stir in the remaining spices and salt. Mix in the peas and the nuts then purée in a blender or food processor until smooth. Turn into a greased ovenproof dish. Drain potatoes and slice fairly thickly. Lay on top of the mixture in the dish in alternate rows with tomato slices.

Brush with the melted butter and either heat through under a moderate preheated grill (broiler) or in a preheated moderate oven (180°C/350°F, Gas Mark 4) for 20 to 30 minutes until the potato is browned.
Serves 4

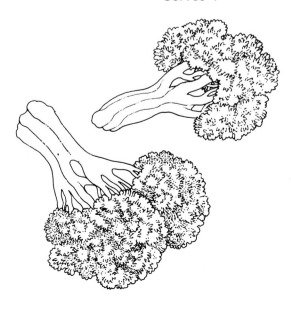

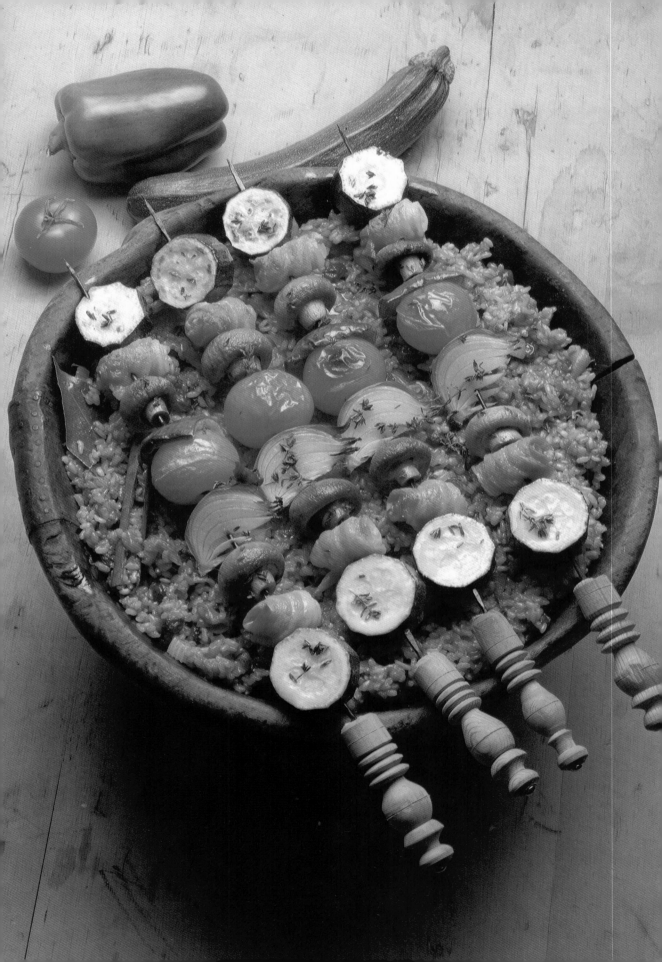

Lunches & Suppers

Bacon Kebabs with Pilaf

METRIC/IMPERIAL
Pilaf:
2 tablespoons oil
1 large onion,
    chopped
2 celery sticks, sliced
225 g/8 oz brown rice
600 ml/1 pint stock
50 g/2 oz seedless
    raisins
50 g/2 oz dried
    apricots, roughly
    chopped
50 g/2 oz walnuts,
    roughly chopped
1 cinnamon stick
1 bay leaf
salt
freshly ground pepper
Kebabs:
225 g/8 oz streaky
    bacon
225 g/8 oz courgettes,
    sliced
8 small tomatoes
1 large onion, cut into
    wedges with skin
8 button mushrooms
1 green pepper, cored,
    seeded and cut into
    8
1 tablespoon oil
1 tablespoon lemon
    juice
1 tablespoon thyme

AMERICAN
Pilaf:
2 tablespoons oil
1 large onion,
    chopped
2 celery stalks, sliced
1 cup brown rice
2½ cups stock
⅓ cup seedless raisins
⅓ cup roughly
    chopped dried
    apricots
½ cup roughly
    chopped walnuts
1 cinnamon stick
1 bay leaf
salt
freshly ground pepper
Kebabs:
½ lb fat bacon slices
1½ cups sliced zucchini
8 small tomatoes
1 large onion, cut into
    wedges with skin
8 button mushrooms
1 green pepper, cored,
    seeded and cut into
    8
1 tablespoon oil
1 tablespoon lemon
    juice
1 tablespoon thyme

To make the pilaf, heat the oil in a pan. Add the onion and celery and fry gently for 5 minutes until golden brown. Add the rice and cook for 1 minute, stirring constantly. Pour on the stock, then add the raisins, apricots and walnuts. Bring to the boil, stirring occasionally, then add the cinnamon, bay leaf and salt and pepper to taste. Lower the heat, cover the pan and simmer for 30 minutes or until the rice is tender and all the stock has been absorbed.

To make the kebabs, remove the rinds then stretch the bacon rashers (slices) with the back of a knife. Cut each rasher (slice) in half then roll up the bacon pieces tightly. Blanch the courgettes (zucchini) in boiling water for 1 minute, then drain. Thread the bacon and vegetables onto 4 large kebab skewers, alternating the different ingredients.

Mix together the oil, lemon juice, thyme and salt and pepper to taste, then brush over the kebabs. Cook on a barbecue or under the grill (broiler) for 5 to 10 minutes until cooked through, turning and basting from time to time.

Spoon the pilaf into a warmed shallow serving dish and arrange the kebabs on top. Serve immediately.
Serves 4

Bacon Kebabs with Pilaf

Chilli Con Carne

METRIC/IMPERIAL	AMERICAN
2 tablespoons cooking oil	2 tablespoons cooking oil
1 onion, sliced	1 onion, sliced
1 clove garlic, crushed	1 clove garlic, crushed
450 g/1 lb minced beef	2 cups ground beef
1 red pepper, cored, seeded and chopped	1 red pepper, cored, seeded and chopped
1 tablespoon chilli powder	1 tablespoon chili powder
2 tablespoons plain flour	2 tablespoons all-purpose flour
300 ml/$\frac{1}{2}$ pint beef stock	1$\frac{1}{4}$ cups beef stock
pinch sugar	pinch sugar
1 × 450 g/16 oz can baked beans	1 × 16 oz can baked beans

Heat the oil in a saucepan and sauté the onion until golden. Add the garlic and the beef and cook, stirring, until the meat is brown. Add the red pepper and cook for a further 3 minutes. Stir in the chilli powder and flour, mix well and then gradually add the beef stock. Bring to the boil, stirring constantly. Cover and cook gently for 30 minutes. Add the sugar and baked beans and cook for a further 10 minutes. Serve with crisp bread and a green salad.
Serves 3 to 4

Potato Chops

METRIC/IMPERIAL	AMERICAN
1 × 450 g/16 oz can baked beans	1 × 16 oz can baked beans
450 g/1 lb potatoes, peeled and sliced	1 lb potatoes, peeled and sliced
salt	salt
freshly ground pepper	freshy ground pepper
4 lamb leg bone steaks	4 lamb leg bone steaks
25 g/1 oz butter, melted	2 tablespoons melted butter
1 tablespoon chopped fresh rosemary	1 tablespoon chopped fresh rosemary

Place the baked beans in the bottom of a greased ovenproof dish. Arrange potato slices on top of the beans steaks and sprinkle with salt and pepper. Place the lamb on top and sprinkle with more salt and pepper.

Mix together the butter and rosemary and spoon over the meat and potatoes. Cover the dish and cook in a preheated moderate oven (180°C/350°F, Gas Mark 4) for 30 minutes. Uncover the dish, increase the oven temperature to hot (220°C/425°F, Gas Mark 7) and cook for a further 15 minutes or until meat and potatoes are tender. Serve hot with baked tomatoes and a green salad.
Serves 4

Beef and Prune Casserole

METRIC/IMPERIAL	AMERICAN
450 g/1 lb stewing beef	1 lb stewing beef
2 tablespoons cooking oil	2 tablespoons cooking oil
1 onion, chopped	1 onion, chopped
1 tablespoon flour	1 tablespoon flour
1 tablespoon tomato purée	1 tablespoon tomato paste
$\frac{1}{4}$ teaspoon mixed herbs	$\frac{1}{4}$ teaspoon mixed herbs
1 × 425 g/15 oz can tomatoes	1 × 16 oz can tomatoes
300 ml/$\frac{1}{2}$ pint red wine or beef stock	1$\frac{1}{4}$ cups red wine or beef stock
225 g/8 oz prunes, soaked in water overnight	1$\frac{1}{3}$ cups prunes, soaked in water overnight
1 × 397 g/14 oz can cannellini beans	1 × 14 oz can cannellini beans
salt	salt
freshly ground pepper	freshly ground pepper
1 tablespoon parsley	1 tablespoon parsley

Trim the meat of excess fat and cut into cubes. Heat the oil in a saucepan and sauté the onion until soft. Add the meat and brown it evenly. Stir in the flour then add the tomato purée (paste), mixed herbs and tomatoes with their juice, and the wine or stock. Bring to the boil, stirring constantly. Add the prunes, cover and simmer gently for about 1$\frac{1}{2}$ hours. Add the drained beans and adjust seasoning to taste. Cook for a further 30 minutes. Sprinkle with parsley and serve with a green salad and baked potatoes.
Serves 4

Spiced Chicken Drumsticks

METRIC/IMPERIAL	AMERICAN
8 chicken drumsticks	8 chicken drumsticks
Coating:	**Coating:**
1 egg	1 egg
1 tablespoon water	1 tablespoon water
4 tablespoons rolled oats	4 tablespoons rolled oats
grated rind of 1 orange	grated rind of 1 orange
1 teaspoon curry powder	1 teaspoon curry powder
1 tablespoon plain flour	1 tablespoon all-purpose flour
50 g/2 oz butter, melted	$\frac{1}{4}$ cup melted butter

Beat the egg with the water. Crush the oats with a rolling pin and mix with the orange rind and curry powder. Coat each drumstick with flour, then egg. Finally pat the oats firmly on to the drumsticks, coating them evenly. Arrange in a roasting pan, pour the melted butter over them and bake in a preheated moderate oven (180°C/350°F, Gas Mark 4) for 20 minutes. Increase the oven temperature to hot (220°C/425°F, Gas Mark 7) and cook the drumsticks for a further 15 minutes or until crisp and golden.

Serve with jacket potatoes or brown rice and green salad.
Serves 4

Shepherd's Squares

METRIC/IMPERIAL	AMERICAN
2 slices brown bread, crumbed	1 cup brown bread crumbs
salt	salt
freshly ground pepper	freshly ground pepper
1 tablespoon made mustard	1 tablespoon prepared mustard
5 tablespoons milk	5 tablespoons milk
450 g/1 lb minced beef	2 cups ground beef
1 × 130 g/5 oz packet instant potato	1 × 130 g package instant potato
2 eggs, beaten	2 eggs beaten
1 small onion, chopped	1 small onion, chopped
1 tablespoon chopped parsley	1 tablespoon chopped parsley
25 g/1 oz butter	2 tablespoons butter
50 g/2 oz Cheddar cheese, grated	$\frac{1}{2}$ cup shredded Cheddar cheese
$\frac{1}{2}$ teaspoon paprika	$\frac{1}{2}$ teaspoon paprika

Combine the breadcrumbs, salt, pepper, mustard and milk and leave to stand until breadcrumbs have softened. Add the minced (ground) meat and mix well. Spread the mixture into a 18 × 28 cm/7 × 11 inch baking pan. Make up the instant potato according to packet instructions. Add the eggs, onion, parsley and seasoning. Spread evenly over the meat mixture and bake in a preheated moderate oven (180°C/350°F, Gas Mark 4) for 35 minutes. Melt the butter and brush over the potato.

Sprinkle with the cheese and paprika and return the pan to the oven for a further 10 minutes. Cut into squares to serve.
Serves 4

Spiced Lamb and Bean Risotto

METRIC/IMPERIAL	AMERICAN
450 g/1 lb shoulder of lamb	1 lb shoulder of lamb
1 onion, chopped	1 onion, chopped
1 clove garlic, crushed	1 clove garlic, crushed
300 ml/$\frac{1}{2}$ pint chicken stock	1$\frac{1}{4}$ cups chicken stock
100 g/4 oz brown sauce	$\frac{1}{2}$ cup brown rice
2 carrots, diced	2 carrots, diced
100 g/4 oz peas	$\frac{2}{3}$ cup peas
2 × 225 g/8 oz cans curried baked beans with sultanas	2 × 8 oz cans curried baked beans with golden raisins
4 tablespoons chopped parsley or mint	4 tablespoons chopped parsley or mint
salt	salt
freshly ground pepper	freshly ground pepper

Cut the meat into small pieces, removing any excess fat. Place in a large saucepan with the onion and garlic and heat gently until the fat begins to run. Increase the temperature and cook, stirring all the time, until the meat colours and the onion softens. Add the stock and rice and simmer gently for 30 minutes, adding more stock if rice looks as though it is going to burn. Add the carrots, peas, curried beans and parsley or mint. Stir well and cook for a further 10 minutes or until meat is tender and rice cooked. Adjust seasoning to taste and serve.
Serves 4

Bacon and Corn Chowder

METRIC/IMPERIAL	AMERICAN
2 tablespoons oil	2 tablespoons oil
100 g/4 oz bacon derinded and chopped	$\frac{1}{4}$ lb bacon, derinded and chopped
2 onions, chopped	2 onions, chopped
1 × 326 g/11$\frac{1}{2}$ oz can sweetcorn	1 × 12 oz can whole kernel corn
50 g/2 oz rolled oats	$\frac{2}{3}$ cup rolled oats
900 ml/1$\frac{1}{2}$ pints chicken stock	3$\frac{3}{4}$ cups chicken stock
1 tablespoon chopped parsley	1 tablespoon chopped parsley
300 ml/$\frac{1}{2}$ pint milk	1$\frac{1}{4}$ cups milk
salt	salt
freshly ground pepper	freshly ground pepper

Heat the oil in a large saucepan and sauté the diced bacon and onion until onion is soft and the bacon cooked. Stir in the corn, oats, stock and parsley. Cover and cook for about 20 minutes, stirring occasionally. Adjust the consistency with the milk if necessary and add seasoning to taste. Heat through and serve.
Serves 4 to 5

Fisherman's Chowder

METRIC/IMPERIAL	AMERICAN
350 g/12 oz potatoes, peeled and sliced	$\frac{3}{4}$ lb potatoes, peeled and thinly sliced
300 ml/$\frac{1}{2}$ pint milk	1$\frac{1}{4}$ cups milk
300 ml/$\frac{1}{2}$ pint water	1$\frac{1}{4}$ cups water
salt	salt
freshly ground pepper	freshly ground pepper
350 g/12 oz whiting fillets, skinned	$\frac{3}{4}$ lb whiting fillets, skinned
4 tablespoons peas	4 tablespoons peas
4 tablespoons sweetcorn	4 tablespoons whole kernel corn
2 tablespoons tomato ketchup	2 tablespoons tomato ketchup
lemon juice to taste	lemon juice to taste

Place the potatoes, milk, water, salt and pepper in a saucepan, cover and simmer gently for 10 minutes. Cut the fish into bite-sized pieces and add to the saucepan with the peas and corn. Simmer, covered, for a further 10 to 15 minutes. Just before serving stir in the tomato ketchup and lemon juice to taste.
Serves 2 to 4

Baked Italian Beans with Bacon

METRIC/IMPERIAL	AMERICAN
225 g/8 oz dried haricot beans	$\frac{1}{2}$ lb dried navy beans
600 ml/1 pint water	2$\frac{1}{2}$ cups water
100 g/4 oz streaky bacon, diced	$\frac{1}{4}$ lb fat bacon, diced
1 onion, peeled and chopped	1 onion, peeled and chopped
1 clove garlic, crushed	1 clove garlic, crushed
1 tablespoon chopped fresh or 1$\frac{1}{2}$ teaspoons dried sage	1 tablespoon chopped fresh or 1$\frac{1}{2}$ teaspoons dried sage
2 tablespoons chopped parsley	2 tablespoons chopped parsley
grated rind and juice of $\frac{1}{2}$ lemon	grated rind and juice of $\frac{1}{2}$ lemon
1 bay leaf	1 bay leaf
salt	salt
freshly ground pepper	freshly ground pepper
1 tablespoon tomato purée	1 tablespoon tomato paste
fresh sage or parsley to garnish	fresh sage or parsley to garnish

Soak the beans in the water overnight. Alternatively cover the beans with 600 ml/1 pint (2$\frac{1}{2}$ cups) boiling water and leave to soak for at least 2 hours.

Heat the oil in a saucepan and fry the bacon, onion and garlic for 5 minutes or until lightly browned. Add the beans with their liquid and all the remaining ingredients. Bring to the boil. Transfer the mixture to a casserole dish, cover and bake in a preheated moderate oven at (180°C/350°F, Gas Mark 4) for 2 to 3 hours or until beans are tender and most of the liquid has been absorbed.

Alternatively cook on top of the cooker in a covered saucepan until the beans are tender, adding a little more water if necessary. Serve hot garnished with sage or parsley.
Serves 4 to 6

Baked Italian Beans with Bacon

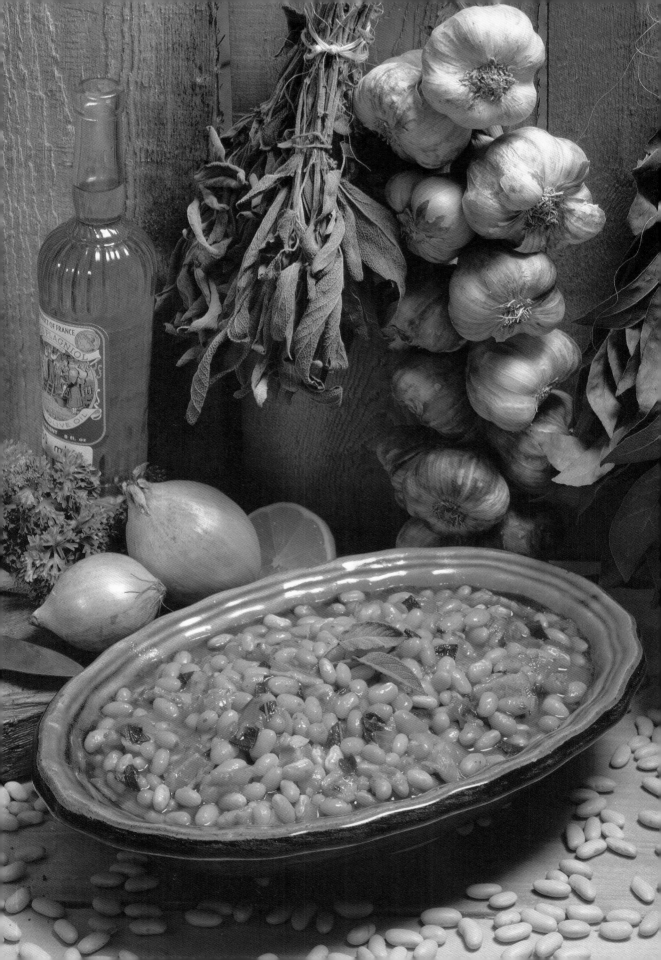

Chicken Casserole

METRIC/IMPERIAL	AMERICAN
2 tablespoons oil	2 tablespoons oil
4 chicken pieces, skinned	1 broiler, cut into 4 and skinned
450 g/1 lb small new potatoes, scrubbed	1 lb small new potatoes, scrubbed
1 onion, chopped	1 onion, chopped
2 carrots, sliced	2 carrots, sliced
250 g/8 oz tomatoes, skinned and chopped	1 cup peeled and chopped tomatoes
100 g/4 oz mushrooms, sliced	1 cup sliced mushrooms
2 tablespoons tomato purée	2 tablespoons tomato paste
50 g/2 oz cornflour	$\frac{1}{3}$ cup cornstarch
600 ml/1 pint chicken stock	$2\frac{1}{2}$ cups chicken stock
4 tablespoons sherry	4 tablespoons sherry
1 × 284 g/10 oz can haricot beans	1 × 10 oz can navy beans
salt	salt
freshly ground pepper	freshly ground pepper
chopped parsley to garnish	chopped parsley to garnish

Heat the oil in a large saucepan and cook the chicken until brown all over. Remove with a slotted spoon and place in a casserole with the potatoes. Add the onion and carrots to the pan and sauté for 5 minutes, then add the tomatoes and mushrooms and cook for a further 2 minutes.

Blend together the tomato purée (paste) and cornflour (cornstarch) and add to the vegetables. Blend in the stock and bring to the boil, stirring, then add the sherry, haricot (navy) beans and salt and pepper to taste.

Pour over the chicken and potatoes, cover and cook in a preheated moderate oven (180°C/350°F, Gas Mark 4) for 1 hour or until the chicken and potatoes are tender. Add a little more stock or water if the casserole is becoming too dry. Serve garnished with parsley.
Serves 4

Chicken and Bean Bake

METRIC/IMPERIAL	AMERICAN
50 g/2 oz butter	4 tablespoons butter
50 g/2 oz flour	$\frac{1}{4}$ cup all-purpose flour
600 ml/1 pint milk	$2\frac{1}{2}$ cups milk
225 g/8 oz cooked chicken, chopped	$\frac{1}{2}$ lb chopped cooked chicken
1 × 450 g/16 oz can baked beans	1 × 16 oz can baked beans
100 g/4 oz pasta shells, cooked	1 cup pasta shells, cooked
100 g/4 oz Cheddar cheese, grated	1 cup shredded Cheddar cheese
2 large tomatoes, sliced	2 large tomatoes, sliced
2 tablespoons flaked almonds	2 tablespoons slivered almonds

Melt the butter in a large saucepan and add the flour. Cook for 2 minutes then remove from heat and gradually stir in the milk. Bring to the boil, stirring constantly. Add the chicken, beans and pasta and two thirds of the cheese. Turn into a well-greased 1 litre/1¾ pint (4 cup) oven-proof dish and top with tomato slices. Sprinkle with remaining cheese and almonds and place under a preheated grill (broiler) until cheese has melted and dish is golden. Alternatively the dish may be left in a cool place until required and then reheated in a preheated moderate oven (180°C/350°F, Gas Mark 4) for 45 minutes.
Serves 3 to 4
Variation:
This dish is also a perfect way of using left over turkey.

Winter Pork and Bean Hot Pot

METRIC/IMPERIAL	AMERICAN
2 tablespoons cooking oil	2 tablespoons cooking oil
1 large onion, chopped	1 large onion, chopped
450 g/1 lb pork, cubed	1 lb pork, cubed
225 g/½ lb carrots, thickly sliced	2 cups thickly sliced carrots
250 ml/8 fl oz chicken stock	1 cup chicken stock
1 × 450 g/16 oz can baked beans	1 × 16 oz can baked beans
Worcestershire sauce	Worcestershire sauce
salt	salt
freshly ground pepper	freshly ground pepper
1 tablespoon chopped parsley	1 tablespoon chopped parsley

Heat the oil in a saucepan and sauté the onion until soft. Add the pork and brown well. Stir in the sliced carrots and chicken stock. Bring to the boil, reduce the heat, cover, and simmer for about 1 hour. Stir in the baked beans and adjust the seasoning to taste with Worcestershire sauce, salt and pepper. Heat for a further 5 minutes and serve sprinkled with parsley.
Serves 4

Broad Bean and Ham Flan

METRIC/IMPERIAL	AMERICAN
225 g/8 oz wholewheat pastry (see page 50)	½ lb wholewheat pastry (see page 50)
40 g/1½ oz butter or margarine	3 tablespoons butter or margarine
25 g/1 oz plain flour	¼ cup all-purpose flour
1 × 284 g/10 oz can broad beans	1 × 10 oz can fava or lima beans
milk	milk
2 tablespoons chopped parsley	2 tablespoons chopped parsley
225 g/8 oz cooked ham, chopped	1 cup cooked diced ham
salt	salt
freshly ground pepper	freshly ground pepper

Roll out the pastry and line a 20 cm (8 inch) flan case. Prick well with a fork and bake blind in a preheated moderately hot oven (200°C/400°F, Gas Mark 6) for 20 to 25 minutes until lightly browned. For the filling, melt the butter in a saucepan, add the flour and cook, stirring for 1 minute. Drain the beans and add enough milk to the liquor from the can to give 300 ml (½ pint). Gradually add this mixture to the flour, stirring well. Bring to the boil, and cook for two minutes. Remove from the heat. Add the beans, parsley, chopped ham and seasoning to taste. Pile into the warm flan case and serve immediately with a salad.
Serves 4 to 6

Sausage and Bean Casserole

METRIC/IMPERIAL	AMERICAN
450 g/1 lb pork sausages	1 lb pork sausages
100 g/4 oz streaky bacon, rind removed and chopped	¼ lb fat bacon, rind removed and chopped
1 large onion, chopped	1 large onion, chopped
2 sticks celery, sliced	2 stalks celery, sliced
1 green pepper, cored, seeded and chopped	1 green pepper, cored, seeded and chopped
2 tablespoons plain flour	2 tablespoons all-purpose flour
500 ml/¾ pint chicken stock	2 cups chicken stock
2 × 425 g/15 oz can kidney beans	2 × 16 oz cans kidney beans
4 carrots, peeled and sliced	4 carrots, peeled and sliced
1 bay leaf	1 bay leaf
salt	salt
freshly ground pepper	freshly ground pepper

Cook the sausages and bacon in a large saucepan over low heat until the fat begins to run then increase the heat and cook until golden. Remove with a slotted spoon and reserve. Add the onion, celery and green pepper to the fat in the saucepan and cook until the onions are translucent. Stir in the flour then gradually add the hot stock. Bring to the boil, stirring constantly. Add kidney beans, carrots, bay leaf, fried bacon and sausage, salt and pepper. Cover the pan and simmer gently for about 30 minutes. Serve with brown rice and a green salad.
Serves 4 to 6

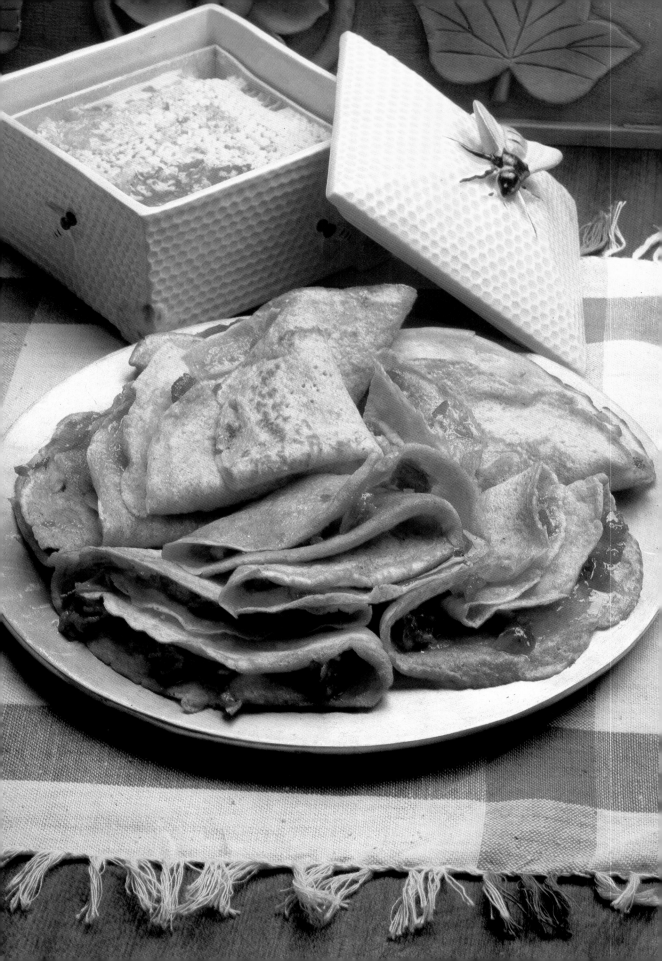

Puddings & Desserts

Wholewheat Crêpes

METRIC/IMPERIAL
100 g/4 oz
   wholewheat self-
   raising flour
1 egg, beaten
300 ml/½ pint milk
2 tablespoons melted
   butter
4 tablespoons clear
   honey
50 g/2 oz seedless
   raisins
pinch of grated
   nutmeg
oil for frying

AMERICAN
1 cup wholewheat
   self-rising flour
1 egg, beaten
1¼ cups milk
2 tablespoons melted
   butter
¼ cup clear honey
⅓ cup seedless raisins
pinch of grated
   nutmeg
oil for frying

Put the flour in a bowl and make a well in the centre. Pour in the egg and milk and beat well to give a smooth batter. Stir in the melted butter. Mix the honey, raisins and nutmeg in a separate bowl.

Heat a little oil in a 20 cm/8 inch frying pan (skillet). When the oil is hot, quickly pour in enough batter to thinly coat the bottom of the pan, tilting the pan to spread the batter evenly. Cook until the top of the batter is set and the underside is golden brown. Turn and cook the other side. Slide onto a warm plate, cover and keep warm by standing the plate over a pan of hot water. Continue until all the batter has been used, making 8 to 10 crêpes in all. Spread each crêpe with a spoonful of the honey mixture then fold to form wedge-shaped parcels.
Serves 4

Wholewheat Crêpes

Prune and Orange Ring

METRIC/IMPERIAL
225 g/8 oz prunes
finely grated rind of 1
   orange
juice of 2 large
   oranges
15 g/½ oz gelatine
juice of 1 lemon
2 egg whites
2 oranges, peel and
   pith removed and
   sliced, to serve

AMERICAN
1⅓ cups prunes
finely grated rind of 1
   orange
juice of 2 large
   oranges
1 envelope unflavored
   gelatin
juice of 1 lemon
2 egg whites
2 oranges, peel and
   pith removed and
   sliced, to serve

Put the prunes and orange rind in a bowl. Make the orange juice up to 300 ml/½ pint/1¼ cups with water, then pour over the prunes. Leave to soak overnight. Alternatively, pour over boiling juice and water and soak for a few hours. Transfer to a pan and bring to the boil. Lower the heat, cover and simmer for 20 minutes until the prunes are tender, then drain, reserving the juice. Measure the juice and make up to 300 ml/½ pint/1¼ cups with water. Remove the stones (seeds) from the prunes. Purée the prune flesh and juice in a blender or food processor.

Sprinkle the gelatine over the lemon juice in a small cup. Stand the cup in a pan of hot water and stir until the gelatine has dissolved. Stir into the prune purée. Beat the egg whites until just stiff, then fold into the mixture. Pour into a 900 ml/1½ pint/3¾ cup ring mould or serving bowl and chill in the refrigerator until set.

To serve, dip the mould in hot water for a few seconds, then invert onto a serving plate. Fill the centre of the ring with the orange slices.
Serves 4 to 6

31

Cheese and Noodle Pudding

METRIC/IMPERIAL	AMERICAN
375 g/12 oz wholewheat noodles	3 cups wholewheat noodles
4 eggs, beaten	4 eggs, beaten
225 g/8 oz cottage cheese	1 cup cottage cheese
150 ml/$\frac{1}{4}$ pint single cream	$\frac{2}{3}$ cup light cream
100 g/4 oz sugar	$\frac{1}{2}$ cup sugar
500 ml/$\frac{3}{4}$ pint milk	2 cups milk
4 tablespoons sultanas	4 tablespoons golden raisins
1$\frac{1}{2}$ teaspoons vanilla essence	1$\frac{1}{2}$ teaspoons vanilla
Topping:	**Topping:**
25 g/1 oz Bran Flakes breakfast cereal	1 cup Bran Flakes breakfast cereal
45 g/1$\frac{1}{2}$ oz butter, melted	3 tablespoons butter, melted
1 tablespoon demerara sugar	1 tablespoon brown sugar
1 teaspoon ground cinnamon	1 teaspoon ground cinnamon

Cook the noodles in boiling water until tender. Drain and rinse thoroughly. Combine the remaining ingredients for the pudding, add to the noodles and mix well. Leave to stand overnight in the refrigerator. Transfer the mixture to a 30 × 20 ml/12 × 8 inch greased baking dish. Bake in a preheated moderate oven (180°C/ 350°F, Gas Mark 4) for 1 hour or until golden. Combine all the ingredients for the topping and spread over the warm pudding.
Serves 4 to 6

Spiced Rhubarb Meringue

METRIC/IMPERIAL	AMERICAN
25 g/1 oz butter or margarine	2 tablespoons butter or margarine
75 g/3 oz sugar	6 tablespoons sugar
2 eggs, separated	2 eggs, separated
75 g/3 oz wholewheat breadcrumbs	1$\frac{1}{2}$ cups wholewheat bread crumbs
1 × 397 g/14 oz can rhubarb	1 × 14 oz can rhubarb
1 teaspoon ground cinnamon	1 teaspoon ground cinnamon

Cream the butter with 2 tablespoons of the sugar. Beat in the egg yolks one at a time. Stir

in the breadcrumbs, rhubarb with its juice and the cinnamon. Transfer the mixture to a greased 1 litre/1$\frac{3}{4}$ pint (4 cup) ovenproof dish. Bake in a preheated moderate oven (180°C/ 350°F, Gas Mark 4) for 15 minutes. Whisk the egg whites until they are very stiff then gradually whisk in the remaining 50 g/2 oz ($\frac{1}{4}$ cup) sugar. Pile this meringue mixture on top of the rhubarb and return to the oven for a further 10 minutes or until meringue is golden.
Serves 4

Tangy Apple Pudding

METRIC/IMPERIAL	AMERICAN
750 g/1$\frac{1}{2}$ lb cooking apples	1$\frac{1}{2}$ lb tart apples
2–3 tablespoons water	2–3 tablespoons water
225 g/8 oz dried apricots, soaked in water	1$\frac{2}{3}$ cups dried apricots, soaked in water
sugar to taste	sugar to taste
Topping:	**Topping:**
75 g/3 oz butter	6 tablespoons butter
100 g/4 oz rolled oats	1$\frac{1}{3}$ cups rolled oats
50 g/2 oz demerara sugar	$\frac{1}{3}$ cup brown sugar
150 ml/$\frac{1}{4}$ pint double cream	$\frac{2}{3}$ cup thick heavy cream
4 tablespoons grated chocolate to decorate	4 tablespoons grated chocolate to decorate

Peel and slice the apples and place in a saucepan with the water and drained apricots. Cook gently until the apricots are soft and apples form a stiff purée. Remove from the heat, add sugar to taste and allow the mixture to cool. For the topping, melt the butter in a frying pan (skillet). Add the rolled oats and cook over a gentle heat for several minutes, stirring constantly. Add the brown sugar, blend thoroughly, then remove from the heat and cool. To assemble the pudding, spoon the fruit mixture into a serving dish and sprinkle the oat mixture on top. Whip the cream until stiff, spoon over the oat mixture and sprinkle with grated chocolate. Serve well chilled.
Serves 4 to 6

Crunchy Apricot Pudding

METRIC/IMPERIAL	AMERICAN
2 × 410 g/15 oz cans apricot halves	2 × 16 oz cans apricot halves
100 g/4 oz butter	½ cup butter
1 teaspoon ground cinnamon	1 teaspoon ground cinnamon
½ teaspoon ground nutmeg	½ teaspoon ground nutmeg
6 tablespoons clear honey	½ cup clear honey
6 slices wholewheat bread	6 slices wholewheat bread
50 g/2 oz Bran Flakes breakfast cereal	2 cups Bran Flakes breakfast cereal
ice cream to serve	ice cream to serve

Drain the apricot halves and reserve 150 ml/¼ pint (⅔ cups) of the syrup. Place the butter, spices and honey into a large saucepan and heat gently. Stir well to mix then stir in the reserved syrup. Remove from the heat. Remove the crusts from the bread, toast until golden on both sides and then cut into 1 cm/½ inch cubes. Add to the butter mixture with the Bran Flakes and the apricot halves. Pour into a 1.5 litre/2½ pint (6 cup) ovenproof dish. Bake in a preheated moderate oven (180°C/350°F, Gas Mark 4) for about 30 minutes. Serve hot or cold with ice cream.
Serves 5 to 6

Apricot Sauce

METRIC/IMPERIAL	AMERICAN
600 ml/1 pint water	2½ cups water
225 g/8 oz dried apricots	1¼ cups dried apricots
300 ml/½ pint sweet white wine	1¼ cups sweet white wine
a few drops of almond essence	a few drops of almond flavoring
about 1 tablespoon lemon juice	about 1 tablespoon lemon juice

Place the water, apricots and wine in a saucepan and bring to the boil. Reduce the heat and simmer gently until the apricots are tender, about 45 minutes. Purée the mixture in a blender or food processor until smooth. Add the almond essence and lemon juice to taste; thin if necessary with white wine or water. Serve hot or cold with ice cream or baked puddings.
Makes 750 ml/1¼ pints (3 cups)

Hot Berry Snow

METRIC/IMPERIAL	AMERICAN
450 g/1 lb mixed red berries (strawberries, raspberries, redcurrants)	3–4 cups mixed red berries (strawberries, raspberries, red currants)
1 tablespoon honey	1 tablespoon honey
150 ml/¼ pint plain yogurt	⅔ cup plain yogurt
2 eggs, separated	2 eggs, separated
1 tablespoon flour	1 tablespoon flour
25 g/1 oz ground almonds	¼ cup ground almonds
2 tablespoons soft brown sugar	2 tablespoons firmly packed light brown sugar

Wash the fruit and place in a baking dish. Spoon over the honey. Put the yogurt in a bowl, then beat in the egg yolks, flour and almonds. Beat the egg whites until stiff, then fold into the yogurt mixture. Spoon over the fruit and sprinkle with the sugar. Bake in a preheated moderately hot oven (200°C/400°F, Gas Mark 6) for 15 to 20 minutes until the topping is risen and golden brown. Serve immediately.
Serves 4

Date and Nut Pudding

METRIC/IMPERIAL	AMERICAN
3 eggs, beaten	3 eggs, beaten
225 g/8 oz sugar	1 cup sugar
4 tablespoons wholewheat flour	4 tablespoons wholewheat flour
1 teaspoon baking powder	1 teaspoon baking powder
450 g/1 lb dates, stones removed and chopped	2½ cups dates, pitted and chopped
100 g/4 oz walnuts, chopped	1 cup chopped walnuts

Beat the eggs and the sugar in a bowl over a pan of boiling water until thick and light. Sift the flour with the baking powder and fold into the egg mixture. Gently stir in the dates and nuts. Pour the mixture into a greased 25 × 20 cm/10 × 8 inch baking pan. Bake in a preheated moderate oven (180°C/350°F, Gas Mark 4) for 30 minutes or until golden. Serve warm topped with whipped cream.
Serves 6 to 8

Hot Fruit Compote

METRIC/IMPERIAL	AMERICAN
175 g/6 oz dried apricots	1 cup dried apricots
450 ml/¾ pint dry cider	2 cups hard cider
3 tablespoons clear honey	3 tablespoons clear honey
150 ml/¼ pint water	⅔ cup water
1 cinnamon stick	1 cinnamon stick
2 cloves	2 cloves
50 g/2 oz seedless raisins	⅓ cup seedless raisins
1 large grapefruit, peel and pith removed and divided into segments	1 large grapefruit, peel and pith removed and divided into segments
2 bananas, peeled and cut into chunks	2 bananas, peeled and cut into chunks

Soak the apricots in the cider for 2 to 3 hours. Place the apricots, cider, honey, water, cinnamon and cloves in a large pan. Bring to the boil, then lower the heat, cover and simmer gently for 15 to 25 minutes, until the apricots are just soft. Add the raisins and simmer for 5 minutes.

Discard the cinnamon stick and cloves. Add the grapefruit segments and banana chunks to the pan and heat through gently. Serve warm, with yogurt if liked.
Serves 4

Spiced Fruit Compote

METRIC/IMPERIAL	AMERICAN
450 g/1 lb mixed dried fruit (apples, apricots, figs, peaches, pears, prunes, sultanas, etc)	3 cups mixed dried fruit (apples, apricots, figs, peaches, pears, prunes, golden raisins, etc)
300 ml/½ pint orange juice	1¼ cups orange juice
300 ml/½ pint water	1¼ cups water
1 cinnamon stick	1 cinnamon stick
2 cloves	2 cloves
50 g/2 oz blanched slivered almonds	½ cup blanched slivered almonds

Put the dried fruit in a bowl and pour over the orange juice and water. Add the spices and leave to soak overnight. Alternatively, pour over boiling juice and water and soak for a few hours.

Transfer to a pan and bring to the boil. Lower the heat, cover and simmer for about 20 minutes or until the fruit is tender, adding more water if the syrup becomes absorbed. Sprinkle with the almonds and serve warm or cold.
Serves 4 to 6

Apricot Syllabub

METRIC/IMPERIAL	AMERICAN
225 g/8 oz dried apricots	1½ cups dried apricots
600 ml/1 pint water	2½ cups water
finely grated rind and juice of 1 lemon	finely grated rind and juice of 1 lemon
150 ml/¼ pint plain yogurt	1¼ cups plain yogurt
2 tablespoons Grand Marnier or other liqueur	2 tablespoons Grand Marnier or other liqueur
50 g/2 oz soft brown sugar	⅓ cup firmly packed light brown sugar
2 egg whites	2 egg whites
lemon twists or chopped nuts to decorate	lemon twists or chopped nuts to decorate

Put the apricots in a bowl, pour over the water, then add the lemon rind and juice. Leave to soak overnight. Alternatively, pour over boiling water with lemon rind and juice and soak for a few hours.

Transfer to a pan and bring to the boil. Lower the heat, cover and simmer for 20 to 30 minutes until the apricots are soft, adding more water if necessary. Work the mixture to a smooth purée in a blender or food processor, then transfer to a bowl and leave to cool.

Stir the yogurt, liqueur and sugar into the purée until well blended. Beat the egg whites until just stiff, then fold into the mixture. Spoon into a serving bowl or 6 individual dishes or glasses, then refrigerate for at least 1 hour before serving. Decorate with lemon twists or nuts.
Serves 6

Apricot Syllabub

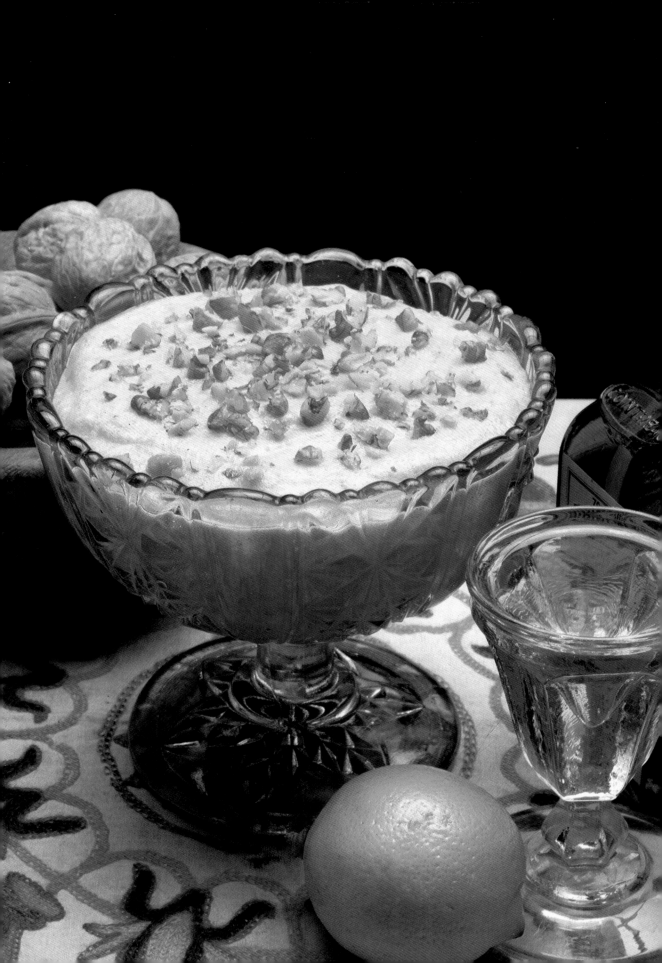

Blackcurrant and Orange Ice Cream

METRIC/IMPERIAL	AMERICAN
225 g/8 oz blackcurrants, stalks removed	2 cups blackcurrants, stalks removed
finely grated rind and juice of 1 orange	finely grated rind and juice of 1 orange
6–8 mint leaves	6–8 mint leaves
4 tablespoons soft brown sugar	$\frac{1}{4}$ cup firmly packed light brown sugar
300 ml/$\frac{1}{2}$ pint plain yogurt	1$\frac{1}{4}$ cups plain yogurt
2 eggs, separated	2 eggs, separated
4–6 small mint sprigs to decorate	4–6 small mint sprigs to decorate

Put the blackcurrants in a blender or food processor, reserving a few for decoration. Add the orange rind and juice, the mint leaves, sugar, yogurt and egg yolks. Blend until smooth. Transfer the purée to a bowl, then place in the freezer, or freezing compartment of the refrigerator. Freeze until half frozen and beginning to thicken.

Beat the egg whites until stiff, then fold into the ice cream. Freeze until half frozen, then beat again to prevent large ice crystals forming, then freeze until firm.

To serve, allow the ice cream to soften slightly at room temperature for about 10 minutes, or in the refrigerator for 20 minutes. Spoon into individual dishes or glasses, then decorate with the reserved blackcurrants and the mint sprigs.
Serves 4 to 6

Bramble Mousse

METRIC/IMPERIAL	AMERICAN
450 g/1 lb blackberries	4 cups blackberries
225 g/8 oz cooking apples, peeled, cored and sliced	1$\frac{1}{2}$ cups peeled, cored and sliced tart apples
finely grated rind and juice of 1 orange or lemon	finely grated rind and juice of 1 orange or lemon
4 tablespoons soft brown sugar	$\frac{1}{4}$ cup firmly packed light brown sugar
15 g/$\frac{1}{2}$ oz gelatine	1 envelope unflavored gelatin
2 tablespoons water	2 tablespoons water
150 ml/$\frac{1}{4}$ pint plain yogurt	$\frac{2}{3}$ cup plain yogurt
2 egg whites	2 egg whites

Put the blackberries in a pan, reserving a few for decoration. Add the apples, orange or lemon rind and juice and the sugar. Cover and heat gently for 10 to 15 minutes until the fruit is soft, stirring occasionally. Rub through a sieve (strainer) into a bowl.

Sprinkle the gelatine over the water in a small cup. Stand the cup in a pan of hot water and stir until the gelatine has dissolved. Stir the gelatine into the fruit purée with the yogurt and mix well. Leave in a cool place until thick and just beginning to set.

Beat the egg whites until just stiff, then fold into the mousse. Transfer to a large serving bowl or individual dishes or glasses. Chill in the refrigerator until set, then decorate with the reserved blackberries. Serve chilled.
Serves 4 to 6

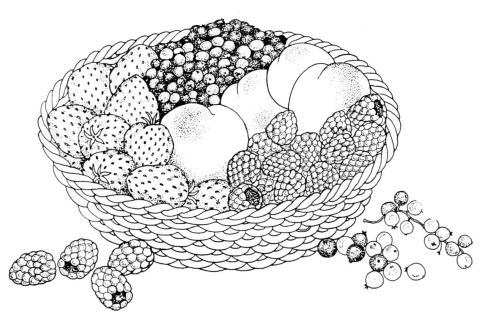

Raspberry Sorbet

METRIC/IMPERIAL	AMERICAN
500 ml/¾ pint water	2 cups water
100 g/4 oz sugar	½ cup sugar
500 ml/¾ pint rosé wine	2 cups rosé wine
450 g/1 lb raspberries	1 lb raspberries
100 ml/4 fl oz lemon juice	½ cup lemon juice
2 tablespoons raspberry liqueur (optional)	2 tablespoons raspberry liqueur (optional)

Place the water and the sugar in a saucepan and heat gently until the sugar has dissolved. Bring the mixture to the boil and boil rapidly for five minutes. Add the wine and the raspberries and simmer until raspberries are soft. Remove from heat, add the lemon juice and the raspberry liqueur if using and purée the mixture in a blender or food processor. Strain through a sieve into a bowl, cover, cool and refrigerate overnight. Taste the mixture, adding more sugar or lemon juice if necessary then transfer it to a metal freezing tray. Cover and freeze until almost solid. Transfer the mixture to the blender or food processor and mix until smooth then refreeze in a covered container. Allow the sorbet to soften a little before serving.
Serves 8

Crumbed Banana and Yogurt Pudding

METRIC/IMPERIAL	AMERICAN
50 g/2 oz butter	4 tablespoons butter
100 g/4 oz wholewheat breadcrumbs	2 cups wholewheat bread crumbs
2 tablespoons demerara sugar	2 tablespoons brown sugar
50 g/2 oz walnuts, chopped	½ cup chopped walnuts
2 large bananas	2 large bananas
juice of 1 lemon	juice of 1 lemon
250 ml/8 fl oz raspberry yogurt	1 cup raspberry yogurt

Melt the butter in a saucepan, remove from heat and stir in the breadcrumbs, sugar and nuts. Allow to cool. Slice the bananas and toss in the lemon juice. Layer the breadcrumb mixture, banana slices and the yogurt in 4 individual glass dishes, or one large glass bowl, ending with a layer of yogurt. Chill thoroughly before serving.
Serves 4
Variation:
Soak 250 g/½ lb prunes in water overnight. Drain and chop them then layer with the above breadcrumb mixture and apricot yogurt instead of raspberry.

Country Trifles

METRIC/IMPERIAL	AMERICAN
1 packet strawberry jelly	1 packet strawberry flavoured gelatin granules
1 × 410 g/15 oz can fruit cocktail	1 × 16 oz fruit cocktail
100 g/4 oz muesli-type breakfast cereal	1 cup Swiss muesli type breakfast cereal
600 ml/1 pint cold custard	2½ cups cold custard
150 ml/¼ pint double cream	⅔ cup heavy cream
Topping:	**Topping:**
2 tablespoons muesli-type breakfast cereal	2 tablespoons Swiss muesli type breakfast cereal
halved glacé cherries	halved glacé cherries

Dissolve the jelly in 150 ml/¼ pint (⅔ cup) boiling water then add it to the syrup from the canned fruit. Make up to 300 ml/½ pint (1¼ cups) with water if necessary. Divide the breakfast cereal into one large or four individual serving dishes. Pour jelly over the cereal and set aside to cool. When jelly has set cover it with the custard and chill. Whip the cream until stiff and pipe it over the custard in decorative swirls. Sprinkle the trifle with the cereal topping and decorate with halved cherries.
Serves 4

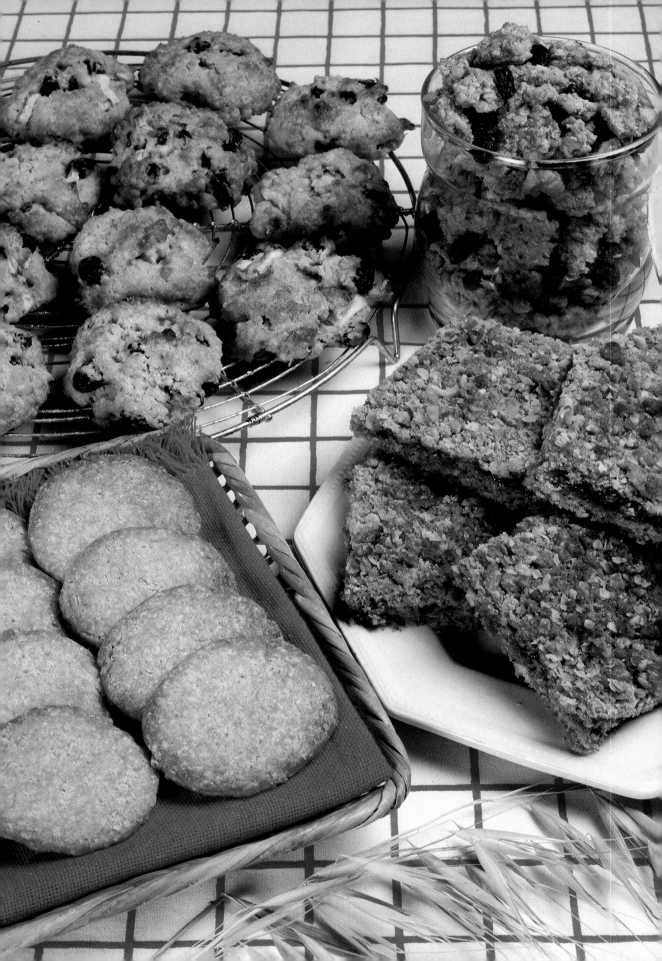

Cakes & Biscuits

Jam Squares

METRIC/IMPERIAL	AMERICAN
175 g/6 oz rolled oats	2 cups rolled oats
225 g/8 oz plain flour	2 cups all-purpose flour
225 g/8 oz butter	1 cup butter
200 g/7 oz soft brown sugar	1 cup firmly packed light brown sugar
50 g/2 oz chopped nuts	$\frac{1}{2}$ cup chopped nuts
1 teaspoon cinnamon	1 teaspoon cinnamon
$\frac{1}{2}$ teaspoon salt	$\frac{1}{2}$ teaspoon salt
$\frac{1}{2}$ teaspoon bicarbonate of soda	$\frac{1}{2}$ teaspoon baking soda
5 tablespoons strawberry jam	5 tablespoons strawberry jam

Place all the ingredients except the jam, in a large bowl. Beat the mixture until it is crumbly. Reserve 500 ml/16 fl oz (2 cups) of the mixture and press the remaining mixture into a well-greased 32 × 23 cm (13 × 9 inch) baking pan. Spread evenly with jam and sprinkle over the reserved mixture. Bake in a preheated hot oven (200°C/400°F, Gas Mark 6) for 30 minutes or until golden. Cool in the pan. Cut into squares to serve.
Makes about 28

Apple and Cheese Pleasers

METRIC/IMPERIAL	AMERICAN
140 g/5$\frac{1}{2}$ oz butter	$\frac{3}{4}$ cup butter
50 g/2 oz soft brown sugar	$\frac{1}{3}$ cup firmly packed light brown sugar
1 egg	1 egg
1 teaspoon vanilla essence	1 teaspoon vanilla extract
75 g/3 oz plain flour	$\frac{3}{4}$ cup all-purpose flour
1 teaspoon ground cinnamon	1 teaspoon ground cinnamon
$\frac{1}{2}$ teaspoon baking powder	$\frac{1}{2}$ teaspoon baking powder
$\frac{1}{2}$ teaspoon salt	$\frac{1}{4}$ teaspon salt
115 g/4$\frac{1}{2}$ oz rolled oats	1$\frac{1}{2}$ cups rolled oats
100 g/4 oz Cheddar cheese, grated	1 cup shredded Cheddar cheese
100 g/4 oz raisins	$\frac{2}{3}$ cup raisins
1 apple, peeled, cored and diced	1 apple, peeled, cored and diced

Cream together the butter and sugar until light. Beat in the egg and vanilla. Sift the flour with the cinnamon, baking powder and salt. Fold into the creamed mixture with the remaining ingredients. Drop heaped teaspoons full of the mixture onto ungreased baking sheets. Bake in a preheated oven (190°C/375°F, Gas Mark 5) for 15 to 20 minutes or until golden. Pack in a tightly covered container and store in the refrigerator.
Makes about 20

Apple and Cheese Pleasers; Snack Crunch (page 7); Jam Squares; Cheese Thins (page 48) (Photograph: Quaker Oats Ltd)

Banana Crunch Cake

METRIC/IMPERIAL	AMERICAN
100 g/4 oz butter or margarine	½ cup butter or margarine
125 g/5 oz demerara sugar	¾ cup brown sugar
225 g/8 oz mashed banana	1 cup mashed banana
2 eggs, beaten	2 eggs, beaten
1 teaspoon vanilla essence	1 teaspoon vanilla
100 g/4 oz oat flour (see Note below)	1 cup oat flour (see Note below)
100 g/4 oz wholewheat flour	1 cup wholewheat flour
1 teaspoon salt	1 teaspoon salt
1 teaspoon bicarbonate of soda	1 teaspoon baking soda
50 g/2 oz walnuts, chopped	½ cup chopped walnuts
Topping:	**Topping:**
50 g/2 oz rolled oats	⅔ cup rolled oats
50 g/2 oz demerara sugar	⅓ cup brown sugar
25 g/1 oz butter, melted	2 tablespoons butter, melted
2 tablespoons chopped walnuts	2 tablespoons chopped walnuts
½ teaspoon ground cinnamon	½ teaspoon ground cinnamon

First make the topping by combining all the ingredients. Mix well and reserve. Beat together the butter and sugar until light and fluffy. Blend in the mashed banana, eggs and vanilla. Mix the dry ingredients then fold into the beaten mixture. Finally fold in the chopped nuts. Pour the mixture into a greased 20 cm/8 inch square baking pan. Sprinkle the crunch topping evenly over the batter. Bake in a preheated moderate oven (180°C/350°F, Gas Mark 4) for about 1 hour or until the cake is golden and a skewer when inserted in the centre of the cake comes out clean. Leave the cake to cool in the tin.

Makes one 1 kg/2 lb cake

Note:
To make oat flour grid rolled oats in a food processor or blender until fine.

Peanut Butter Dreams

METRIC/IMPERIAL	AMERICAN
225 g/8 oz butter	1 cup butter
225 g/8 oz peanut butter	1 cup peanut butter
100 g/4 oz sugar	½ cup sugar
175 g/6 oz demerara sugar	1 cup brown sugar
2 eggs, beaten	2 eggs, beaten
1 teaspoon vanilla essence	1 teaspoon vanilla
275 g/9 oz oat flour (see Note for previous recipe)	2¼ cups ground oat flour (see Note for previous recipe)
2 teaspoons bicarbonate of soda	2 teaspoons baking soda
½ teaspoon salt	½ teaspoon salt
125 g/5 oz peanuts (dry roasted), chopped	1 cup chopped peanuts (dry roasted)

Beat together the butter, peanut butter, white and brown sugars until light and fluffy. Gradually beat in the egg followed by the vanilla. Combine all the dry ingredients then stir into the butter mixture. Fold in the nuts. Chill the mixture for about 1 hour then shape into 2 to 3 cm/1 inch balls. Place these balls well apart on an ungreased baking sheet. Flatten with the tines of a fork dipped in sugar to form a criss-cross pattern. Bake in a preheated moderate oven (180°C/350°F, Gas Mark 4) for about 15 minutes or until the edges turn golden. Cool on a wire rack.

Makes about 65

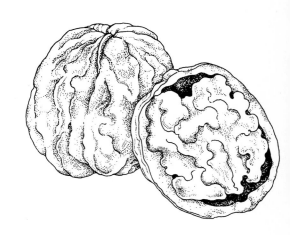

Country Cake

METRIC/IMPERIAL	AMERICAN
100 g/4 oz butter or margarine	$\frac{1}{2}$ cup butter or margarine
100 g/4 oz sugar	$\frac{1}{2}$ cup sugar
grated rind of $\frac{1}{2}$ lemon	grated rind of $\frac{1}{2}$ lemon
2 eggs, beaten	2 eggs, beaten
50 g/2 oz self-raising flour	$\frac{1}{2}$ cup self-rising flour
$\frac{1}{2}$ teaspoon baking powder	$\frac{1}{2}$ teaspoon baking powder
50 g/2 oz wholewheat flour	$\frac{1}{2}$ cup wholewheat flour
125 g/5 oz muesli-type breakfast cereal	$1\frac{1}{2}$ cups Swiss muesli style breakfast cereal
150 ml/$\frac{1}{4}$ pint	$\frac{2}{3}$ cup milk

Cream together the butter and sugar until light and fluffy. Beat in the lemon rind followed by the eggs. Sift the self-raising flour with the baking powder and fold into the mixture with a metal spoon. Add the wholewheat flour, the breakfast cereal and enough milk to give a soft dropping consistency. Pour the mixture into a greased and lined 1 kg/2 lb loaf pan and bake in a preheated moderate oven (180°C/350°F, Gas Mark 4) for about 50 minutes or until the cake is golden and a skewer inserted in the centre comes out clean. Transfer to a wire rack to cool.
Makes one 1 kg/2 lb cake

Honey Crisps

METRIC/IMPERIAL	AMERICAN
100 g/4 oz butter or margarine	$\frac{1}{2}$ cup butter or margarine
100 g/4 oz demerara sugar	$\frac{2}{3}$ cup demerara brown sugar
75 g/3 oz honey	$\frac{1}{4}$ cup honey
275 g/9 oz wholewheat flour	$2\frac{1}{4}$ cups wholewheat flour
$\frac{1}{2}$ teaspoon ground ginger	$\frac{1}{2}$ teaspoon ground ginger
$\frac{1}{2}$ teaspoon ground cinnamon	$\frac{1}{2}$ teaspoon ground cinnamon
$\frac{1}{4}$ teaspoon bicarbonate of soda	$\frac{1}{4}$ teaspoon baking soda

Beat together the butter or margarine, sugar and honey until the mixture is light and fluffy. Stir in the remaining ingredients, mixing well. (The dough will be stiff and dry.) Shape a teaspoonful of the dough into a ball and place on an ungreased baking sheet. Continue until all the mixture is used. Bake in a preheated moderately hot oven (190°C/375°F, Gas Mark 5) for 10 to 12 minutes. Allow to cool on the baking sheet for 1 minute and then transfer to a wire cooling rack. Store in an airtight container.
Makes about 36

Coconut Snowballs

METRIC/IMPERIAL	AMERICAN
100 g/4 oz rolled oats	1 cup rolled oats
100 g/4 oz wholewheat flour	1 cup wholewheat flour
75 g/3 oz ground almonds	$\frac{3}{4}$ cup ground almonds
25 g/1 oz icing sugar	$\frac{1}{4}$ cup icing sugar
100 g/4 oz butter	$\frac{1}{2}$ cup butter
few drops almond essence	few drops almond extract
Coating:	**Coating:**
40 g/1$\frac{1}{2}$ oz desiccated coconut	$\frac{1}{2}$ cup desiccated coconut
$1\frac{1}{2}$ tablespoons icing sugar	$1\frac{1}{2}$ tablespoons icing sugar

Stir together the oats, flour and ground almonds. Sift the icing sugar into a bowl. Add the butter and almond essence (extract) and cream together until light and fluffy. Fold in the oat mixture, mixing thoroughly. The dough will be rather sticky at this stage, so allow it to stand in the refrigerator for about 15 minutes. Shape into 36 to 40 small balls. Spread the coconut on to a flat dish and roll the balls in the coconut until well coated. Place on an ungreased baking sheet allowing about 3 cm/1$\frac{1}{2}$ inches between the balls. Bake in a preheated moderate oven (180°C/350°F, Gas Mark 4) for about 15 minutes.

Cool on the baking sheet for 5 minutes then transfer the biscuits (cookies) to a wire cooling rack. When cold sift the icing sugar over the balls.
Makes 36 to 40

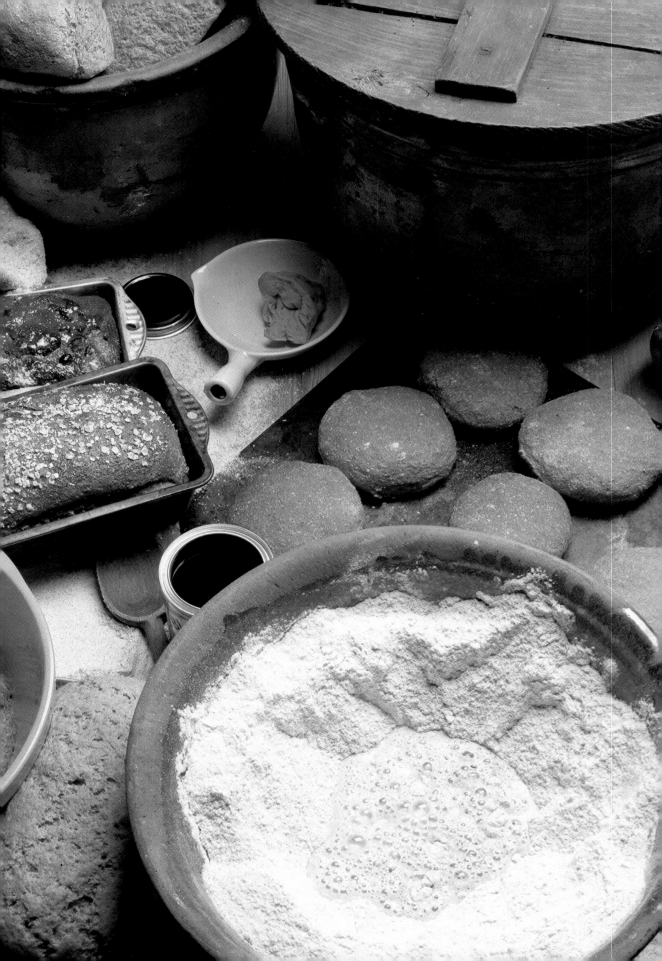

Savoury Breads Pastries & Pies

Farmhouse Bread

METRIC/IMPERIAL	AMERICAN
1.5 kg/3 lb wholewheat flour	12 cups wholewheat flour
25 g/1 oz sea salt	1 tablespoon coarse salt
25 g/1 oz Muscovado sugar	1½ tablespoons Barbados sugar
25 g/1 oz fresh yeast	1 cake compressed yeast
900 ml/1½ pints lukewarm water	3¾ cups lukewarm water
1 tablespoon vegetable oil	1 tablespoon vegetable oil
beaten egg to glaze	beaten egg to glaze

Put the flour, salt and sugar in a warm bowl and mix well. Blend the yeast with a little of the water, then stir into the remaining water and add to the dry ingredients with the oil. Mix to a soft dough. Turn out onto a lightly floured surface and knead for 5 minutes until smooth. Place the dough in a warm, greased bowl. Cover with a damp cloth and leave in a warm place for about 1 hour until doubled in size.

Turn out onto the floured surface and knead again for 5 minutes, then divide the dough into 4 pieces. Fold each piece into 3, then place in greased, warmed 450 g/1 lb loaf tins (pans). Cover with a damp cloth and leave in a warm place for about 30 minutes until the dough rises to the tops of the tins (pans).

Brush the dough with beaten egg, then bake in a preheated hot oven (230°C/450°F, Gas Mark 8) for 40 minutes. Turn out onto a wire rack and leave to cool.
Makes four 450 g/1 lb loaves

A selection of breads made using wholewheat flour

Rich Bran Loaf

METRIC/IMPERIAL	AMERICAN
100 g/4 oz All Bran breakfast cereal	1 cup All Bran breakfast cereal
100 g/4 oz soft brown sugar	⅔ cup firmly packed light brown sugar
50 g/2 oz raisins	⅓ cup raisins
50 g/2 oz sultanas	⅓ cup golden raisins
100 g/4 oz dried figs, chopped	⅔ cup dried figs, chopped
300 ml/½ pint milk	1¼ cups milk
100 g/4 oz self-raising flour	1 cup self-rising flour

Place the All Bran, sugar, dried fruit and milk into a bowl. Mix well and leave to stand for ½ hour. Sift in the flour and mix well with a metal spoon. Turn the batter into a greased and lined 1 kg/2 lb loaf tin (pan) and bake in a preheated moderate oven (180°C/350°F, Gas Mark 4) for about 1 hour. Turn out on to wire rack and leave to cool. Serve sliced with butter.
Makes one 1 kg/2 lb loaf

Buttermilk Bran Muffins

METRIC/IMPERIAL	AMERICAN
100 g/4 oz unprocessed bran	2 cups unprocessed bran
100 g/4 oz plain flour	1 cup all-purpose flour
1 teaspoon baking powder	1 teaspoon baking powder
pinch salt	pinch salt
300 ml/½ pint buttermilk	1¼ cups buttermilk
1 egg, beaten	1 egg, beaten
4 tablespoons raisins	4 tablespoons raisins
2 tablespoons clear honey	2 tablespoons honey
3 tablespoons black treacle	2 tablespoons molasses

In a large bowl mix together bran, flour, baking powder and salt. Stir in the remaining ingredients and stir until just combined. Do not overmix. Spoon into paper-cup-lined muffin pans, filling them two-thirds full. Bake in a preheated moderately hot oven (190°C/375°F, Gas Mark 5) for about 25 minutes or until golden and a skewer when inserted comes out clean. Serve warm with butter.
Makes about 15

Oat and Raisin Bread

METRIC/IMPERIAL	AMERICAN
150 g/5 oz plain flour	1¼ cups all-purpose flour
1 tablespoon baking powder	1 tablespoon baking powder
pinch salt	pinch salt
1 teaspoon ground cinnamon	1 teaspoon ground cinnamon
½ teaspoon ground nutmeg	½ teaspoon ground nutmeg
100 g/4 oz rolled oats	1⅓ cup rolled oats
175 g/6 oz demerara sugar	1 cup brown sugar
150 g/5 oz wholewheat flour	1¼ cups wholewheat flour
300 ml/½ pint milk	1¼ cups milk
2 eggs, beaten	2 eggs, beaten
6 tablespoons cooking oil	6 tablespoons cooking oil
175 g/6 oz raisins	1 cup raisins
50 g/2 oz walnuts, chopped	½ cup chopped walnuts
1 tablespoon grated orange rind	1 tablespoon grated orange rind

Sift the plain (all-purpose) flour, baking powder, salt and spices into a large bowl. Add the oats, sugar and wholewheat flour, mix well. Add the milk, eggs and oil and mix until the dry ingredients are just moistened. Stir in the raisins, nuts and orange rind. Do not over mix. Spoon into a greased and floured 1 kg/2 lb loaf tin (pan) and bake in a preheated moderate oven (180°C/350°F, Gas Mark 4) for about 1¼ hours or until a skewer inserted in the centre of the cake comes out clean. Cool in the pan for 10 minutes then turn out on to a wire rack. Serve sliced and buttered.
Makes one 1 kg/2 lb loaf

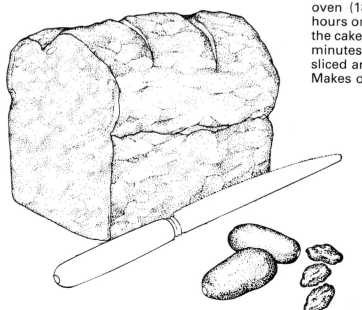

Mocha Flapjacks

METRIC/IMPERIAL	AMERICAN
50 g/2 oz butter	$\frac{1}{4}$ cup butter
2 tablespoons golden syrup	2 tablespoons golden syrup
2 teaspoons coffee essence	2 teaspoons coffee flavoring
50 g/2 oz plain chocolate, roughly chopped	2 squares semi-sweet chocolate, roughly chopped
4 tablespoons chopped walnuts	4 tablespoons chopped walnuts
100 g/4 oz rolled oats	1 cup rolled oats

Heat the butter and syrup in a small saucepan until the butter has melted. Stir in the coffee essence, chocolate, nuts and oats and mix well. Spread the mixture into a lightly greased 17–18 cm/7 inch square baking pan and cook in a preheated moderate oven (160°C/325°F, Gas Mark 3) for 25–30 minutes. Cut into fingers while warm but allow the flapjacks to cool in the pan before removing.
Makes 12

Crunchy Bars

METRIC/IMPERIAL	AMERICAN
450 g/1 lb rolled oats	4 cups rolled oats
150 g/6 oz nuts, chopped	1$\frac{1}{2}$ cups chopped nuts
225 g/8 oz soft brown sugar	1$\frac{1}{3}$ cups firmly packed light brown sugar
175 g/6 oz butter or margarine, melted	$\frac{3}{4}$ cup butter or margarine, melted
175 g/6 oz clear honey	$\frac{1}{2}$ cup honey
1 teaspoon vanilla essence	1 teaspoon vanilla
pinch salt	pinch salt

Place all the ingredients in a large bowl and mix well. Press the mixture into a well-greased square 23–25 cm/9–10 inch roasting pan and bake in a preheated very hot oven (230°C/450°F, Gas Mark 8) for 10 to 12 minutes or until golden brown and bubbly. Cool in the tin before cutting into bars.
Makes 25

Oatmeal Gingerbread

METRIC/IMPERIAL	AMERICAN
150 g/5 oz plain flour	1$\frac{1}{4}$ cups all-purpose flour
pinch of salt	pinch of salt
1 tablespoon ground ginger	1 tablespoon ground ginger
1 teaspoon ground cinnamon	1 teaspoon ground cinnamon
2 teaspoons baking powder	2 teaspoons baking powder
150 g/5 oz rolled oats	1$\frac{2}{3}$ cups rolled oats
175 g/6 oz soft brown sugar	1 cup firmly packed light brown sugar
6 tablespoons black treacle	6 tablespoons molasses
100 g/4 oz butter or margarine	$\frac{1}{2}$ cup butter or margarine
1 egg, beaten	1 egg, beaten
250 ml/8 fl oz milk	1 cup milk
100 g/4 oz sultanas	$\frac{2}{3}$ cup golden raisins
50 g/2 oz blanched almonds, roughly chopped	$\frac{1}{2}$ cup roughly chopped blanched almonds

Sift the flour, salt, spices and baking powder into a mixing bowl and stir in the oats and sugar. Warm the treacle (molasses) and margarine in a small saucepan until margarine has melted. Stir well then add to the bowl with the egg and milk. Beat well until smooth. Stir in the sultanas and nuts and spoon the mixture into a square 18 cm/7 inch cake tin that has been lined with greaseproof (waxed) paper. Bake in a preheated moderate oven (180°C/350°F, Gas Mark 4) for 1$\frac{1}{4}$ hours or until a skewer inserted in the centre comes out clean. Allow cake to cool in the tin. Cut into squares.
Serves 6 to 8

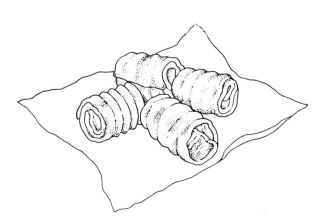

Date and Nut Loaf

METRIC/IMPERIAL	AMERICAN
175 g/6 oz plain flour	1½ cups all-purpose flour
2½ teaspoons baking powder	2½ teaspoons baking powder
½ teaspoon ground cinnamon	½ teaspoon ground cinnamon
¼ teaspoon ground nutmeg	¼ teaspoon ground nutmeg
pinch of salt	pinch of salt
175 g/6 oz wholewheat flour	1½ cups wholewheat flour
175 g/6 oz soft brown sugar	1 cup firmly packed light brown sugar
100 g/4 oz rolled oats	1⅓ cups rolled oats
250 ml/8 fl oz plain yogurt or soured cream	1 cup plain yogurt or sour cream
120 ml/4 fl oz corn oil	½ cup corn oil
3 tablespoons milk	3 tablespoons milk
2 eggs	2 eggs
175 g/6 oz dates, stoned	1 cup pitted dates
100 g/4 oz walnuts, roughly chopped	1 cup walnuts, roughly chopped

Sift the plain flour, baking powder, spices and salt into a mixing bowl. Stir in the wholewheat flour, sugar and rolled oats. Mix thoroughly. Beat together the yogurt, oil, milk and eggs. Add to the flour mixture and beat thoroughly. Fold in the dates and nuts and mix thoroughly. Spoon the mixture into two greased 1 kg/2 lb loaf tins and bake in a preheated moderate oven (180°C/350°F, Gas Mark 4) for about 1 hour or until a skewer inserted in the centre comes out clean. Leave the loaves in the pans for 5 minutes then turn out on to a wire rack to cool completely.
Makes two 1 kg/2 lb loaves
Note:
This loaf freezes well.

Fruit Malt Loaf

METRIC/IMPERIAL	AMERICAN
225 g/8 oz wholewheat flour	2 cups wholewheat flour
100 g/4 oz sultanas	¾ cup golden raisins
25 g/1 oz vegetable margarine	2 tablespoons vegetable margarine
50 g/2 oz malt extract	3 tablespoons malt extract
25 g/1 oz black treacle	1½ tablespoons molasses
25 g/1 oz fresh yeast	1 cake compressed yeast
75 ml/2½ fl oz lukewarm water	⅓ cup lukewarm water
1 tablespoon clear honey to glaze	1 tablespoon honey to glaze

Put the flour and sultanas (golden raisins) in a warm bowl and mix well. Put the margarine, malt extract and black treacle (molasses) in a pan and heat gently until the margarine has melted. Leave to cool for 5 minutes.

Blend the yeast with the water, then add to the dry ingredients with the melted mixture. Mix to a soft dough. Turn out onto a lightly floured surface and knead for 5 minutes until smooth. Place the dough in a warmed, greased bowl. Cover and leave in a warm place for about 1 hour until doubled in size.

Turn out onto the floured surface and knead again for 5 minutes. Fold the dough into 3, then place in a greased, warmed 450 g/1 lb loaf tin. Cover with a clean damp cloth and leave in a warm place for about 20 minutes until the dough rises to the top of the tin.

Bake in a preheated moderately hot oven (200°C/400°F, Gas Mark 6) for 45 minutes. Turn out onto a wire rack, brush with honey, then leave to cool.
Makes one 450 g/1 lb loaf

Fruit Malt Loaf

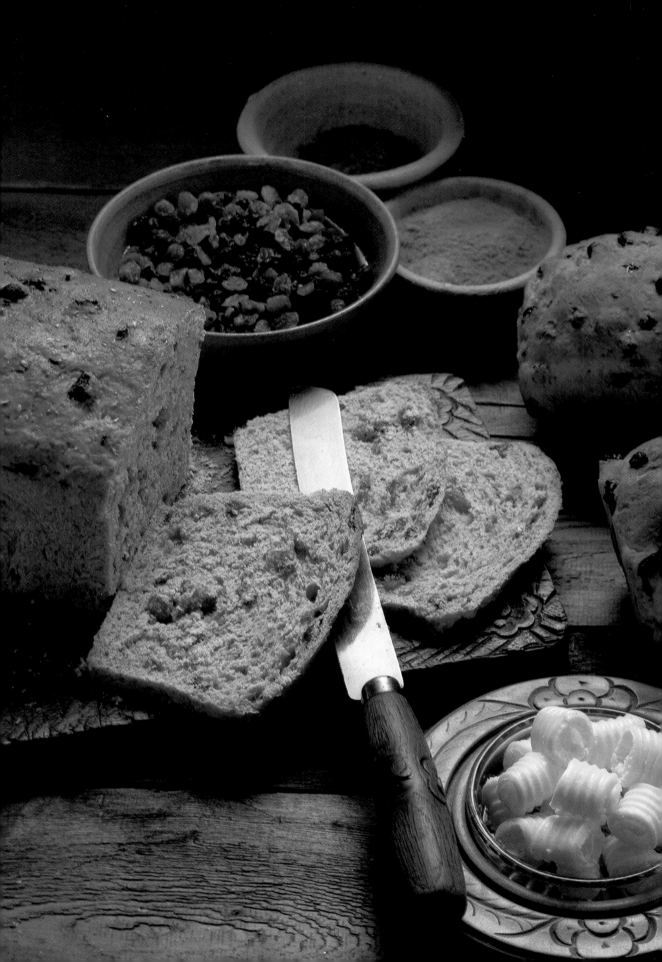

Cheese Crackers

METRIC/IMPERIAL
225 g/8 oz Cheddar
  cheese, grated
50 g/2 oz grated
  Parmesan cheese
125 g/4 oz butter
3 tablespoons water
150 g/5 oz plain flour
½ teaspoon mustard
  powder
pinch salt
75 g/3 oz rolled oats

AMERICAN
2 cups shredded
  Cheddar cheese
½ cup grated
  Parmesan cheese
½ cup butter
3 tablespoons water
1¼ cups all-purpose
  flour
½ teaspoon mustard
  powder
pinch salt
1 cup rolled oats

Beat together the cheeses, butter and water until well blended. Sift together the flour, mustard and salt and fold into the cheese mixture followed by the rolled oats. Shape the dough into a roll about 30 cm/12 inches long. Wrap securely in foil or greaseproof (waxed) paper and refrigerate for about 4 hours. Uncover and cut the roll into 5 mm/¼ inch slices and transfer to a greased baking sheet. Flatten slightly with a fork then bake in a preheated hot oven (200°C/400°F, Gas Mark 6) for 8 to 10 minutes or until the edges are light golden. Transfer to a wire rack and allow to cool.
Makes about 60

Cheese Thins

METRIC/IMPERIAL
125 g/4 oz rolled oats
½ teaspoon mustard
  powder
¼ teaspoon cayenne
  pepper
50 g/2 oz butter
75 g/3 oz Cheddar
  cheese, grated
¼ teaspoon
  bicarbonate of soda
2 tablespoons boiling
  water

AMERICAN
1⅓ cups rolled oats
½ teaspoon dry
  mustard
¼ teaspoon cayenne
4 tablespoons butter
¾ cup shredded
  Cheddar cheese
¼ teaspoon baking
  soda
2 tablespoons boiling
  water

Mix together the rolled oats, mustard and cayenne. Rub (cut) in the butter then stir in the grated cheese. Dissolve the soda in the boiling water and pour over the dry ingredients. Mix to a stiff consistency adding a little extra water if necessary. Turn out on to a floured board and knead lightly. Roll out the mixture until it is about 5 mm/¼ inch thick. Cut into rounds using a 7 cm/2½-3 inch biscuit cutter. Transfer the rounds to a greased baking sheet and bake in a preheated moderately hot oven (190°C/375°F, Gas Mark 5) for about 10 minutes or until golden. Transfer to a wire rack to cool.
Makes about 20

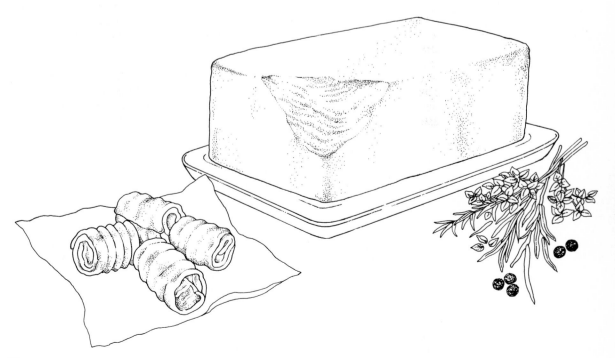

Wholewheat Cheese Pastry

METRIC/IMPERIAL	AMERICAN
150 g/6 oz wholewheat flour	1½ cups wholewheat flour
pinch of salt	pinch of salt
½ teaspoon mustard powder	½ teaspoon dry mustard
pinch cayenne pepper	pinch cayenne
75 g/3 oz butter or margarine	6 tablespoons butter or margarine
75 g/3 oz Cheddar cheese, finely grated	¾ cup shredded Cheddar cheese
2 tablespoons cold water	2 tablespoons cold water

Mix together the flour, salt, mustard and cayenne in a large mixing bowl. Rub (cut) in the fat until the mixture resembles breadcrumbs. Mix in the grated (shredded) cheese. Add the water and using a knife cut the mixture until it comes together to form a dough. Use your hands to knead lightly. Chill for 30 minutes before using for pies, pasties or to line savoury flan cases.

Herbed Bread Round

METRIC/IMPERIAL	AMERICAN
225 g/8 oz plain flour	2 cups all-purpose flour
225 g/8 oz wholewheat flour	2 cups wholewheat flour
½ teaspoon salt	½ teaspoon salt
1 teaspoon bicarbonate of soda	1 teaspoon baking soda
25 g/1 oz butter	2 tablespoons butter
2 large onions, grated	2 cups shredded onion
3 sticks celery, sliced	3 stalks celery, sliced
1 teaspoon dried mixed herbs	1 teaspoon dried mixed herbs
2 tablespoons chopped parsley	2 tablespoons chopped parsley
250 ml/8 fl oz buttermilk or plain yogurt	1 cup buttermilk or plain yogurt
a little milk to glaze	a little milk to glaze

Combine the flours, salt and soda in a large mixing bowl. Rub (cut) in the butter then stir in the onion, celery and herbs. Mix well. Add enough of the buttermilk to give a soft dough. Turn out on to a lightly floured surface and knead lightly. Shape into a 22 cm/9 inch round and place on a floured baking sheet. Score the top into 8 segments and brush with milk. Bake in a preheated hot oven (200°C/400°F, Gas Mark 6) for 30 to 35 minutes or until well risen and golden. Serve warm with soups, salads or cheese.
Serves 8

Sultana Spice Biscuits

METRIC/IMPERIAL	AMERICAN
100 g/4 oz butter	½ cup butter
175 g/6 oz soft brown sugar	⅞ cup firmly packed light brown sugar
50 g/2 oz mashed potato, sieved	¼ cup sieved mashed potato
175 g/6 oz wholewheat flour	1½ cups wholewheat flour
50 g/2 oz sultanas	⅓ cup golden raisins
1 teaspoon mixed spice	1 teaspoon mixed spice
Topping:	**Topping:**
1 tablespoon caster sugar	1 tablespoon sugar
½ teaspoon mixed spice	½ teaspoon mixed spice

Cream together the butter and sugar until smooth and fluffy, then beat in the potato.

Add the flour, sultanas (golden raisins) and spice and mix well. Turn on to a lightly floured surface and roll out to 5 mm/¼ inch thick. Using a 7 cm/2½ inch cutter, cut out rounds and place them on greased baking sheets.

Bake in a preheated moderate oven (180°C/350°F, Gas Mark 4) for 15 to 20 minutes until golden brown. Mix together the sugar and spice and sprinkle over the hot biscuits. Transfer to a wire rack and allow to cool.
Makes about 20

Wholewheat Pastry

METRIC/IMPERIAL	AMERICAN
100 g/4 oz plain flour	1 cup all-purpose flour
100 g/4 oz wholewheat flour	1 cup wholewheat flour
pinch of salt	pinch of salt
100 g/4 oz butter or margarine	½ cup butter or margarine
2 egg yolks	2 egg yolks
1 tablespoon cold water	1 tablespoon cold water

Place the flours and salt in a mixing bowl then rub (cut) in the butter or margarine until the mixture resembles fine breadcrumbs. Beat the egg yolks with the water then add to the dry mixture and mix to a dough. Cover and chill before using.

Note:

This pastry can be made using all wholewheat flour but it is then more difficult to handle and it is best to roll it out on a piece of foil so that it can be easily lifted.

Wholewheat Mortadella Scones

METRIC/IMPERIAL	AMERICAN
100 g/4 oz self-raising flour	1 cup self-rising flour
100 g/4 oz wholewheat flour	1 cup wholewheat flour
1½ teaspoons baking powder	1½ teaspoons baking powder
50 g/2 oz butter	¼ cup butter
50 g/2 oz Mortadella sausage, diced	¼ cup diced Mortadella sausage
150 ml/¼ pint milk	⅔ cup milk

Mix the flours and baking powder together. Rub (cut) in the butter and mix in the Mortadella. Pour in the milk and mix lightly to form a fairly soft dough. Roll out on a lightly floured surface to 1 cm/½ inch thickness.

Using a 5 cm/2 inch cutter, cut out approximately 12 scones. Place on a greased baking sheet and brush with milk. Place in a preheated hot oven (220°C/425°F, Gas Mark 7) and bake for 10 to 12 minutes. Serve warm.

Makes 12

Focaccia

METRIC/IMPERIAL	AMERICAN
25 g/1 oz fresh yeast, or 15 g/½ oz dried yeast	1 cake compressed yeast, or 1 tablespoon dried yeast
1 teaspoon sugar	1 teaspoon sugar
450 ml/¾ pint warm water	2 cups warm water
450 g/1 lb strong plain white flour	4 cups strong all-purpose white flour
450 g/1 lb wholewheat flour	4 cups wholewheat flour
salt	salt
150 ml/¼ pint olive oil	⅔ cup olive oil
3 onions, thinly sliced	3 onions, thinly sliced
1 egg	1 egg
100 g/4 oz black olives	¾ cup ripe olives

Add the fresh or dried yeast to 150 ml/¼ pint (⅔ cup) warm water with the sugar. Leave the yeast in a warm place for 10 minutes until frothy.

Sieve 225 g/8 oz (2 cups) white flour into a bowl with the salt. Make a well in the centre and pour in the yeast mixture and 3 tablespoons oil. Mix to a soft dough. Knead on a lightly floured surface for 5 minutes. Place dough in a large oiled polythene bag and leave in a warm place for 1 hour until doubled in size.

Meanwhile, heat 3 tablespoons oil and sauté onion for 5 minutes until soft. allow to cool.

When the dough has doubled in size, sieve the remaining flour into a separate bowl, make a well in the centre and add the egg, remaining 4 tablespoons oil and remaining 300 ml/½ pint (1⅓ cups) warm water. Mix well together then add the risen dough. Turn out onto a floured board and knead for 5 minutes. Return to the oiled bag and leave to rise for 45 minutes.

Divide dough in half. Roll to a 5 mm/¼ inch thickness and use to line two baking sheets 30 × 23 cm/12 × 9 inches. Spread over the cooked onions and oil. Add the olives and brush generously with extra oil. Place in a preheated hot oven (220°C/425°F, Gas Mark 7) and bake for 30 minutes. Serve hot or cold.

Makes 16 slices

Focaccia; Wholewheat Mortadella Scones

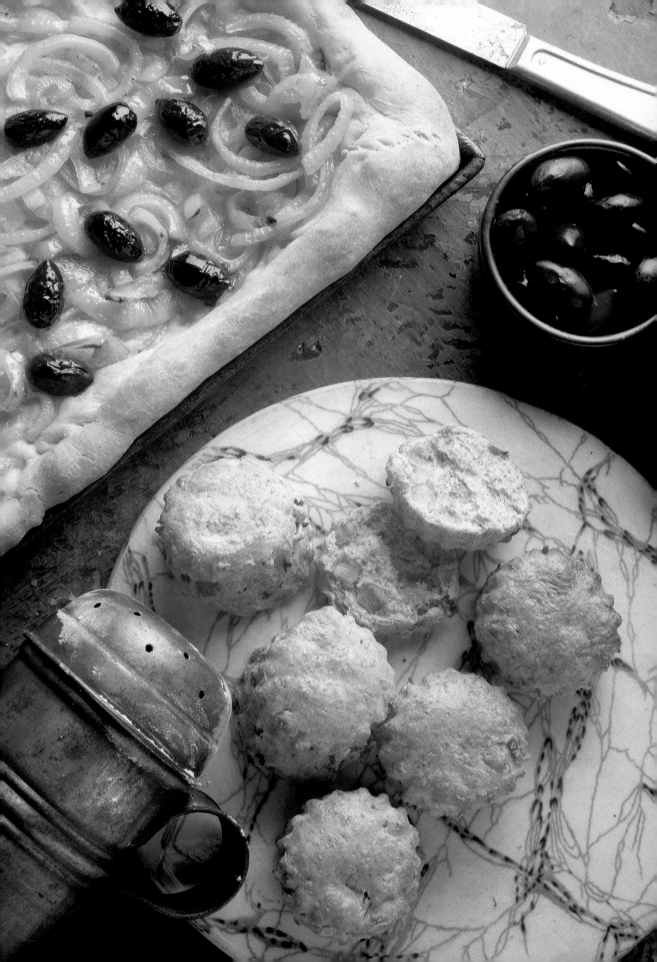

Nutty Leek and Egg Pie

METRIC/IMPERIAL	AMERICAN
1 quantity wholewheat pastry (see page 50)	1 quantity wholewheat pastry (see page 50)
milk to glaze	milk to glaze
Filling:	**Filling:**
25 g/1 oz butter	2 tablespoons butter
2 tablespoons cooking oil	2 tablespoons cooking oil
500 g/1 lb leeks, sliced	1 lb leeks, sliced
25 g/1 oz flour	2 tablespoons flour
300 ml/½ pint milk	1¼ cups milk
1 chicken stock cube	2 chicken bouillon cubes
100 g/4 oz Cheddar cheese, grated	1 cup shredded Cheddar cheese
4 tablespoons peanuts or cashews, chopped	4 tablespoons peanuts or cashews, chopped
4 hard-boiled eggs, sliced	4 hard-cooked eggs, sliced
salt	salt
freshly ground pepper	freshly ground pepper

For the filling, heat the butter and oil in a large saucepan. Add the leeks, stir thoroughly then cover and leave to cook gently for about 10 minutes or until the leeks are soft. Stir in the flour then gradually add the milk. Add the stock (bouillon) cube, bring to the boil, stirring constantly. Remove from the heat and add the cheese, nuts, eggs, salt and pepper. Turn the mixture into a well-greased 1 litre/1¾ pint (4 cup) ovenproof pie dish.

Roll out the pastry until about 5 mm/¼ inch thick. Cut a long strip about 1 cm/½ inch wide and lay around the edge of the pie dish, moistened with a little water. Moisten the pastry strip and lay the rolled out pastry on top. Trim the edges and crimp the edges with a knife to seal. Decorate the top of the pie with pastry leaves cut from pastry trimmings. Glaze the pie with milk and bake in a preheated hot oven (200°C/400°F, Gas Mark 6) for 25 to 30 minutes or until the pastry is lightly browned.
Serves 4 to 6

Individual Farmhouse Pies

METRIC/IMPERIAL	AMERICAN
1 quantity wholewheat pastry (see page 50)	1 quantity wholewheat pastry (see page 50)
milk to glaze	milk to glaze
Filling:	**Filling:**
1 small onion, chopped	1 small onion, chopped
2 sticks celery, sliced	2 stalks celery, sliced
25 g/2 oz butter	¼ cup butter
1 tablespoon flour	1 tablespoon all-purpose flour
150 ml/¼ pint milk	⅔ cup milk
175 g/6 oz cooked chicken, chopped	¾ cup chopped cooked chicken
1 × 225 g/8 oz can baked beans	1 × 8 oz can baked beans
salt	salt
freshly ground pepper	freshly ground pepper
½ teaspoon oregano	½ teaspoon oregano

For the filling sauté the onion and the celery in the butter until the onion is transparent. Stir in the flour and cook for 1 minute. Gradually add the milk, stirring well. Bring to the boil and cook for 1 minute. Remove from the heat, add the chicken, baked beans, seasoning and oregano and leave to cool. Roll out two thirds of the wholewheat pastry and use to line four individual 10 cm/4 inch patty pans leaving a generous edge of pastry. Spoon in prepared filling. Roll out remaining pastry, cut into 10 cm/4 inch rounds and place on top of filling. Moisten the top and bottom edges with water and press together to seal well. Make a slash in the top of each pie to allow the steam to escape. Brush the pastry with a little milk and bake in a preheated hot oven (200°C/400°F, Gas Mark 6) for 25 to 30 minutes until pastry is golden. Serve warm or cold with a selection of salads. Makes 4

Corn and Pepper Stuffing

METRIC/IMPERIAL	AMERICAN
50 g/2 oz butter	¼ cup butter
1 onion, chopped	1 onion, chopped
1 × 326 g/11½ oz can sweetcorn, drained	1 × 12 oz can whole kernel corn, drained
2 red peppers, cored, seeded and chopped	2 red peppers, cored, seeded and chopped
grated rind of 1 lemon	grated rind of 1 lemon
50 g/2 oz wholewheat breadcrumbs	1 cup wholewheat bread crumbs
salt	salt
freshly ground pepper	freshly ground pepper
1 egg, beaten	1 egg, beaten

Melt the butter in a saucepan and gently sauté the onion until soft but not coloured. Add the drained corn, peppers, lemon rind and breadcrumbs. Add salt and pepper then bind the mixture with the egg.
Sufficient for a 2½ kg/5 lb turkey

Sausage and Raisin Stuffing

METRIC/IMPERIAL	AMERICAN
60 g/2 oz seedless raisins	⅓ cup seedless raisins
75 g/3 oz butter	6 tablespoons butter
3 sticks celery, sliced	3 stalks celery, sliced
225 g/8 oz sausage meat	½ lb sausage mince
50 g/2 oz wholewheat breadcrumbs	1 cup wholewheat bread crumbs
1 egg, beaten	1 egg, beaten
salt	salt
freshly ground pepper	freshly ground pepper

Place the raisins in a bowl and pour over sufficient boiling water to cover. Leave to stand for 5 minutes then drain and dry. Melt the butter in a saucepan and sauté the sliced celery without browning it. Remove from the heat and cool slightly. Mix the sausage meat (mince), breadcrumbs, raisins, and celery. Bind the mixture with the egg and season well with salt and pepper.
Sufficient to stuff a 3 kg/6 lb bird

Spiced Carrot Chews

METRIC/IMPERIAL	AMERICAN
150 g/5 oz plain flour	1¼ cups all-purpose flour
1 teaspoon baking powder	1 teaspoon baking powder
pinch of salt	pinch of salt
1 teaspoon ground cinnamon	1 teaspoon ground cinnamon
¼ teaspoon ground nutmeg	¼ teaspoon ground nutmeg
¼ teaspoon ground cloves	¼ teaspoon ground cloves
225 g/8 oz margarine	1 cup margarine
175 g/6 oz soft brown sugar	1 cup firmly packed light brown sugar
1 egg, beaten	1 egg, beaten
1 teaspoon vanilla essence	1 teaspoon vanilla
225 g/8 oz rolled oats	2 cups rolled oats
6 carrots, grated	2 cups shredded carrots
50 g/2 oz chopped nuts	½ cup chopped nuts
75 g/3 oz raisins	½ cup raisins

Sift together the flour, baking powder, salt and spices. In a large bowl beat together the margarine and sugar until the mixture is light and fluffy. Blend in the egg and vanilla. Using a metal spoon fold in the flour mixture followed by the oats, carrot, nuts and raisins. Drop rounded tablespoons of the mixture on to a greased baking sheet and bake in a preheated moderate oven (180°C/350°F, Gas Mark 4) for 13 to 15 minutes. Cool for a minute on the baking sheet and then transfer the biscuits to a wire rack.
Makes about 30

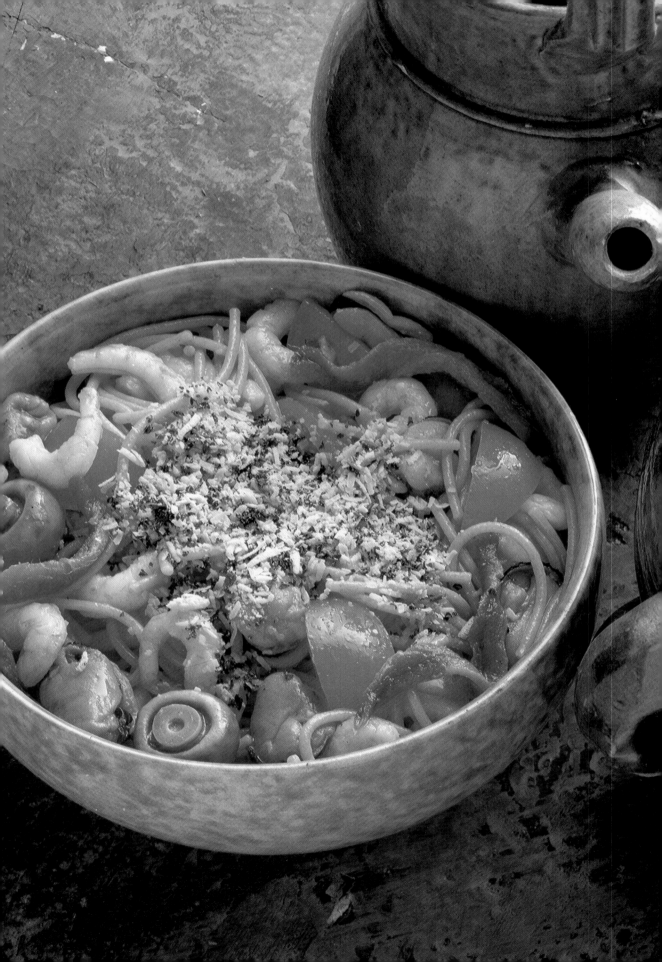

High Fibre Salads

Sardinian Seafood Salad

METRIC/IMPERIAL
225 g/8 oz wholewheat
  macaroni
salt
25 g/1 oz butter
50 g/2 oz mushrooms
100 g/4 oz cooked and
  shelled mussels
100 g/4 oz peeled
  prawns
1 × 50 g/1¾ oz can
  anchovies, drained
3 tomatoes, cut into
  wedges
Dressing:
5 tablespoons olive oil
1 tablespoon lemon
  juice
1 tablespoon wine
  vinegar
1 clove garlic, crushed
salt
freshly ground pepper
½ teaspoon dried
  oregano
To garnish:
2 tablespoons
  chopped parsley
2 tablespoons grated
  Parmesan cheese
4 lemon twists

AMERICAN
½ lb wholewheat
  macaroni
salt
2 tablespoons butter
2 oz mushrooms
½ cup cooked and
  shelled mussels
⅔ cup shelled shrimp
1 × 2 oz can
  anchovies, drained
3 tomatoes, cut into
  wedges
Dressing:
5 tablespoons olive oil
1 tablespoon lemon
  juice
1 tablespoon wine
  vinegar
1 clove garlic, crushed
salt
freshly ground pepper
½ teaspoon dried
  oregano
To garnish:
2 tablespoons
  chopped parsley
2 tablespoons grated
  Parmesan cheese
4 lemon twists

First, make the dressing: mix together the oil, lemon juice, vinegar, garlic and salt and pepper to taste. Add the oregano. Allow the dressing to stand for 1 hour for the flavours to blend.

Cook the macaroni in a large pan of boiling salted water for 10 minutes until tender but *al dente*. Drain thoroughly.

Meanwhile, melt the butter in a small pan, add the mushrooms and sauté for 3 minutes. Drain on kitchen paper towels. While still warm, mix the pasta with the mussels, prawns (shrimp) and anchovies. Add the mushrooms and tomatoes and pour over the dressing. Mix thoroughly and turn into a serving dish. Chill in the refrigerator for 2 hours.

Sprinkle over the chopped parsley and Parmesan cheese and garnish with lemon twists. Serve immediately.
Serves 4 to 6

Piquant Bean Salad

METRIC/IMPERIAL
1 × 200 g/7½ oz can red
  kidney beans
1 × 284 g/10 oz can
  butter beans
4 sticks celery, sliced
4 gherkins, sliced
1 tablespoons capers
  (optional)
sliced cucumber to
  garnish
3 tablespoons
  mayonnaise

AMERICAN
1 × 8 oz can red kidney
  beans
1 × 10 oz can navy
  beans
4 stalks celery, sliced
4 gherkins, sliced
1 tablespoon capers
  (optional)
sliced cucumber to
  garnish
3 tablespoons
  mayonnaise

Drain the beans and mix with the sliced celery, gherkins, and capers. Arrange the cucumber slices around the edge of an oval serving dish. Pile the bean mixture in the centre and trickle the mayonnaise over the top.
Serves 2 to 4

Sardinian Seafood Salad

Egg and Kidney Bean Salad

METRIC/IMPERIAL
440 g/15½ oz can red
 kidney beans
4 tablespoons
 chopped parsley
1 onion, chopped
salt
freshly ground pepper
2 hard-boiled eggs,
 sliced
2 tomatoes, thinly
 sliced
Dressing:
a pinch each of salt,
 pepper, mustard
 powder and sugar
2 tablespoons salad
 oil
1 tablespoon red wine
 vinegar
1 teaspoon
 Worcestershire
 sauce
sprig of parsley for
 garnish

AMERICAN
1 × 16 oz can red
 kidney beans
4 tablespoons
 chopped parsley
1 onion, chopped
salt
freshly ground pepper
2 hard-cooked eggs,
 sliced
2 tomatoes, thinly
 sliced
Dressing:
a pinch each of salt,
 pepper, dry
 mustard and sugar
2 tablespoons salad
 oil
1 tablespoon red wine
 vinegar
1 teaspoon
 Worcestershire
 sauce
sprig of parsley for
 garnish

Drain the beans well and place in a serving dish. Mix in the chopped parsley. Peel the onion, slice off a couple of thin rings and put to one side. Finely chop the remainder and add to the beans. Season with salt and pepper. Beat the dressing ingredients together and stir into the beans. Garnish the dish with the egg and tomato slices and decorate with the reserved onion rings and parsley.
Serves 3 to 4

Three Bean Salad

METRIC/IMPERIAL
1 × 450 g/16 oz can
 baked beans
1 × 450 g/16 oz can red
 kidney beans
175 g/6 oz French
 beans, lightly
 cooked
1 onion, chopped
1 clove garlic, crushed
1 teaspoon made
 mustard
4 tablespoons olive oil
1 tablespoon white
 wine vinegar
salt
freshly ground pepper
2 hard-boiled eggs,
 chopped
2 tablespoons
 chopped parsley

AMERICAN
1 × 16 oz can baked
 beans
1 × 16 oz can red
 kidney beans
1½ cups green beans,
 lightly cooked
1 onion, chopped
1 clove garlic, crushed
1 teaspoon prepared
 mustard
4 tablespoons olive oil
1 tablespoon white
 wine vinegar
salt
freshly ground pepper
2 hard-cooked eggs,
 chopped
2 tablespoons
 chopped parsley

Drain the baked beans, reserving the "juice". Mix the baked beans with the drained kidney beans, French (green) beans and the onion. Blend the bean "juice" with the garlic, mustard, oil, vinegar and seasoning to taste. Spoon this dressing over the beans and mix well. Carefully stir in the chopped eggs and serve sprinkled with parsley.
Serves 6

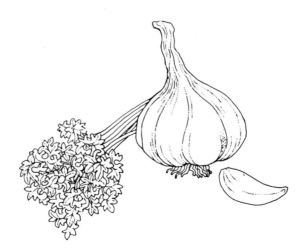

Toast and Bean Salad

METRIC/IMPERIAL	AMERICAN
4 slices wholewheat bread	4 slices wholewheat bread
75 g/3 oz Cheddar cheese, grated	¾ cup shredded Cheddar cheese
1 lettuce, shredded	1 lettuce, shredded
4 spring onions, chopped	4 scallions, chopped
3 sticks, celery, sliced	3 stalks celery, sliced
1 × 450 g/16 oz can red kidney beans, drained	1 × 16 oz can red kidney beans, drained
150 g/6 oz cooked ham, diced	¾ cup cooked diced ham
4 tablespoons vinaigrette dressing (see page 62)	4 tablespoons French dressing (see page 62)
2 tablespoons chopped parsley	2 tablespoons chopped parsley

Remove the crusts from the bread and toast on both sides. Sprinkle one side with cheese and place under a preheated grill until the cheese has melted. Cut the toasted bread into 1 cm/½ inch squares. Place shredded lettuce into a serving bowl and pile the onions (scallions), celery, drained beans and ham on top. Just before serving, pour over the dressing and toss well. Sprinkle with toasted bread cubes and parsley and serve.
Serves 4

Chinese Salad

METRIC/IMPERIAL	AMERICAN
225 g/8 oz bean sprouts	2 cups bean sprouts
¼ cucumber, chopped	1 cup chopped cucumber
8 radishes, sliced	8 radishes, sliced
4 spring onions, chopped	4 scallions, chopped
1 × 450 g/16 oz can baked beans	1 × 16 oz can baked beans
1 apple, cored and sliced	1 apple, cored and sliced
1 carrot, grated	1 carrot, shredded
8 stoned dates, chopped	8 pitted dates, chopped
225 g/8 oz cooked ham, diced	1 cup diced cooked ham
watercress to garnish	watercress to garnish
Dressing:	**Dressing:**
4 tablespoons white wine vinegar	4 tablespoons white wine vinegar
1 tablespoon soy sauce	1 tablespoon soy sauce
2 tablespoons clear honey	2 tablespoons clear honey
pinch mustard powder	pinch dry mustard
salt	salt
freshly ground pepper	freshly ground pepper

Place all the ingredients for the salad in a large bowl and mix well. For the dressing, place the ingredients in a small screw-top jar and shake thoroughly to mix. Pour the dressing over the salad and toss well so that the ingredients are well coated. Turn the salad on to a serving dish. Garnish with watercress and serve.
Serves 4

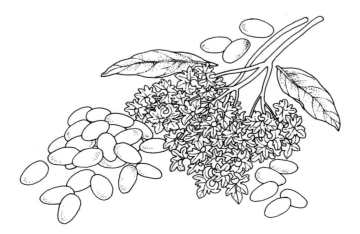

Brown Rice Salad with Yogurt Dressing

METRIC/IMPERIAL	AMERICAN
225 g/8 oz brown rice, cooked	1 cup brown rice, cooked
2 tomatoes, chopped	2 tomatoes, chopped
2 small courgettes, grated	2 small zucchini, shredded
1 green pepper, cored, seeded and chopped	1 green pepper, cored, seeded and chopped
2 carrots, grated	2 carrots, shredded
1 × 326 g/11½ oz can sweetcorn, drained	1 × 12 oz can whole kernel corn, drained
225 g/8 oz frozen peas, cooked	1½ cups frozen peas, cooked
Dressing:	*Dressing:*
250 ml/8 fl oz plain yogurt	1 cup plain yogurt
4 tablespoons lemon juice	4 tablespoons lemon juice
grated rind of 1 lemon	grated rind of 1 lemon
3 tablespoons salad oil	3 tablespoons salad oil
½ teaspoon dried basil or 1 tablespoon fresh	½ teaspoon dried basil or 1 tablespoon fresh
1 clove garlic, crushed	1 clove garlic, crushed
salt	salt
freshly ground pepper	freshly ground pepper

Mix all the ingredients for the salad in a large bowl. For the dressing, beat together all the ingredients and pour over the rice salad. Toss lightly and serve.
Serves 4 to 6

Orange Salad

METRIC/IMPERIAL	AMERICAN
4 oranges	4 oranges
1 × 425 g/15 oz can red kidney beans	1 × 16 oz can red kidney beans
225 g/8 oz bean sprouts	2 cups bean sprouts
4 sticks celery, sliced	4 stalks celery, sliced
2 tablespoons well seasoned vinaigrette dressing (see page 62)	2 tablespoons well seasoned French dressing (see page 62)
1 tablespoon chopped parsley	1 tablespoon chopped parsley

Using a sharp knife remove the peel and pith from the oranges and cut into segments free of any membrane. Retain any juice. Drain the beans well and place in a bowl with the orange segments, any retained orange juice, bean sprouts and celery. Add the dressing and parsley and toss well.
Serves 4 to 6

Orange and Watercress Salad

METRIC/IMPERIAL	AMERICAN
1 large bunch watercress, trimmed	1 large bunch watercress, trimmed
3 oranges, peel and pith removed and thinly sliced into rounds	3 oranges, peel and pith removed and thinly sliced into rounds
1 onion, thinly sliced	1 onion, thinly sliced
1 small green pepper, cored, seeded and thinly sliced	1 small green pepper, cored, seeded and thinly sliced
6 tablespoons vinaigrette dressing (see page 62)	6 tablespoons French dressing (see page 62)
black olives to garnish	ripe olives to garnish

Put the watercress in a salad bowl. Arrange the orange slices on top with the onion and pepper rings. Pour on the dressing and garnish with the olives. Serve chilled.
Serves 4

Orange Salad
(Photograph: Summer Orange Office)

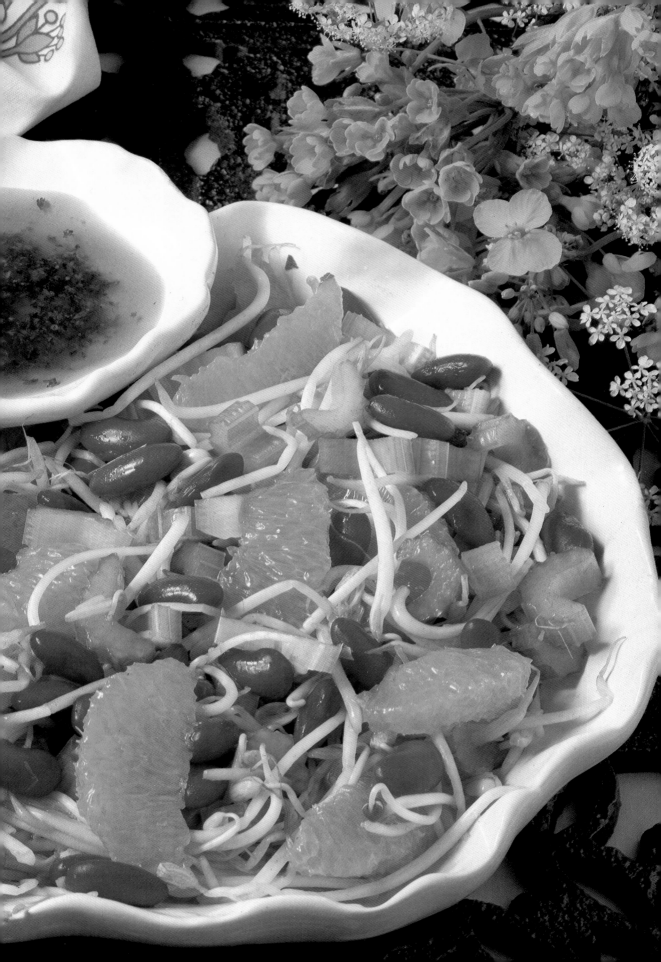

Creamy Bean Salad

METRIC/IMPERIAL
1 × 200 g/7½ oz red
  kidney beans
1 × 284 g/10 oz can
  broad beans
1 × 225 g/8 oz can
  black eyed beans
4 tomatoes, peeled
  and chopped
2 cloves garlic,
  crushed
1 teaspoon caraway
  seeds
2 teaspoons tomato
  purée
120 ml/4 fl oz
  mayonnaise
salt
freshly ground pepper

AMERICAN
1 × 8 oz can red kidney
  beans
1 × 10 oz can lima
  beans
1 × 8 oz black eyed
  beans
4 tomatoes, peeled
  and chopped
2 cloves garlic,
  crushed
1 teaspoon caraway
  seeds
2 teaspoons tomato
  paste
½ cup mayonnaise
salt
freshly ground pepper

Drain the canned beans and place in a large
bowl with the tomatoes, garlic and caraway
seeds. Mix well. Blend together the tomato
purée (paste), mayonnaise, salt and pepper.
Pour over the vegetable mixture and stir
thoroughly. Chill before serving.
Serves 4 to 6

Ham and Pineapple Pasta Salad

METRIC/IMPERIAL
225 g/8 oz
  wholewheat pasta
225 g/8 oz cooked
  ham, diced
1 × 284 g/10 oz can
  pineapple pieces,
  drained
100 g/4 oz peas,
  cooked
150 ml/¼ pint plain
  yogurt
1 tablespoon lemon
  juice
1 tablespoon chopped
  chives
salt
freshly ground pepper

AMERICAN
2 cups wholewheat
  pasta
1 cup diced cooked
  ham
1 × 10 oz can
  pineapple pieces,
  drained
½ cup peas, cooked
⅔ cup plain yogurt
1 tablespoon lemon
  juice
1 tablespoon chopped
  chives
salt
freshly ground pepper

Cook the pasta in plenty of boiling salted water
until tender. Drain and rinse with cold water.
Transfer the pasta to a large bowl and allow to
cool completely. Add the chopped ham,
drained pineapple and peas. Mix well. Combine
the yogurt, lemon juice, chopped chives, salt
and pepper to taste. Add to the pasta mixture
and toss thoroughly before serving.
Serves 4

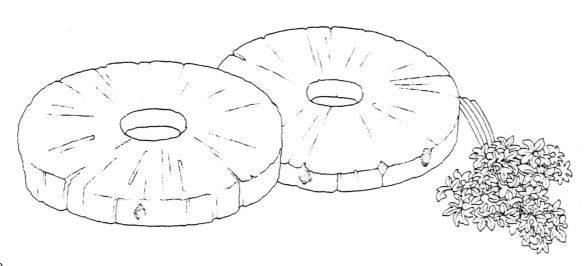

Brown Rice Salad

METRIC/IMPERIAL	AMERICAN
100 g/4 oz brown rice	½ cup brown rice
salt	salt
100 g/4 oz shelled peas or sliced French beans	¾ cup shelled peas, or ½ cup sliced green beans
100 g/4 oz sweetcorn	¾ cup whole kernel corn
150 ml/¼ pint vinaigrette dressing (see page 62)	⅔ cup French dressing (see page 62)
1 red pepper, cored, seeded and diced	1 red pepper, cored, seeded and diced
50 g/2 oz salted peanuts	½ cup salted peanuts
1 small onion, grated	1 small onion, shredded
freshly ground pepper	freshly ground pepper

Cook the rice in boiling salted water for 30 minutes or until tender. Add the peas or beans and corn and simmer for a further few minutes until just tender. Drain thoroughly.

Transfer to a bowl and add half of the dressing while the rice and vegetables are still hot. Toss well to mix, then leave to cool. Add the remaining ingredients and dressing and mix well. Taste and adjust the seasoning just before serving. Serve cold.
Serves 4

Citrus Chicken and Spinach Salad

METRIC/IMPERIAL	AMERICAN
450 g/1 lb cooked chicken	2 cups cooked chicken
450 g/1 lb spinach	1 lb spinach
2 oranges	2 oranges
1 leek, finely sliced	1 leek, finely sliced
4 tablespoons chopped walnuts	4 tablespoons chopped walnuts
Dressing:	**Dressing:**
150 ml/¼ pint salad oil	⅔ cup salad oil
juice of 1 lemon	juice of 1 lemon
2 cloves garlic, crushed	2 cloves garlic, crushed
salt	salt
freshly ground pepper	freshly ground pepper

Cut the chicken into strips. Wash the spinach, dry it well then tear into bite-sized strips. Remove the peel and white pith from the oranges and cut the segments from the membrane. Wash and dry the sliced leek. For the dressing, combine all the ingredients and pour over the chicken. Marinate for several hours in a cool place. To serve the salad, toss together the spinach, orange segments, leek and chicken together with the marinade. Transfer to a salad bowl and sprinkle with the chopped walnuts.
Serves 4
Variation:
Omit the walnuts and sprinkle over 2 rashers (slices) bacon that has been cooked until crisp and then crumbled.

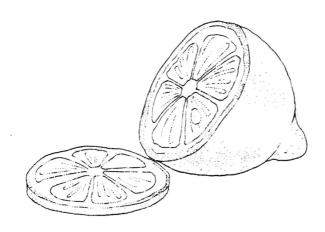

Butter Bean Vinaigrette

METRIC/IMPERIAL
2 × 284 g/10 oz cans
  butter beans,
  drained
1 large onion
120 ml/4 fl oz salad oil
4 tablespoons white
  wine vinegar
1 clove garlic
salt
freshly ground pepper
¼ teaspoon nutmeg
½ teaspoon made
  mustard
2 tablespoons freshly
  chopped parsley

AMERICAN
2 × 10 oz cans lima
  beans, drained
1 large onion
½ cup salad oil
¼ cup white wine
  vinegar
1 clove garlic
salt
freshly ground pepper
¼ teaspoon ground
  nutmeg
½ teaspoon prepared
  mustard
2 tablespoons freshly
  chopped parsley

Place the well-drained beans into a bowl. Peel
the onion and cut into very thin rings. Add to
the beans. Mix the salad oil with the vinegar.
Crush the garlic with the salt and add to the oil
mixture with the seasoning, nutmeg and mustard. Beat thoroughly then pour over the beans
and toss well. Leave to stand for at least 1 hour
before serving sprinkled with parsley.
Serves 4

Vinaigrette (French) Dressing

METRIC/IMPERIAL
150 ml/¼ pint oil
5 tablespoons wine
  vinegar or lemon
  juice
1 clove garlic, crushed
salt
freshly ground pepper
pinch of sugar
¼ teaspoon mustard
  powder
1 teaspoon chopped
  fresh herbs of your
  choice or ½ teaspoon
  dried

AMERICAN
⅔ cup oil
5 tablespoons wine
  vinegar or lemon
  juice
1 clove garlic, crushed
salt
freshly ground pepper
pinch of sugar
¼ teaspoon dry
  mustard
1 teaspoon chopped
  fresh herbs of your
  choice or ½ teaspoon
  dried

Place all the ingredients in a screw-topped jar.
Shake well. Store in the refrigerator and use
when required, shaking well before use.
Makes about 175 ml/6 fl oz (¾ cup)

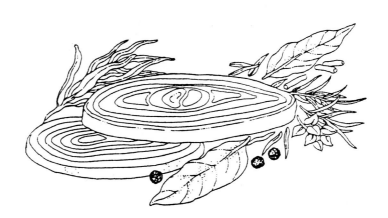

Index

Acknowledgements

The publishers would like to thank Quaker and Scotts Porage Oats for
their co-operation and acknowledge the following photographers:
Robert Golden 51, 54; Gina Harris 26, 47; Roger Phillips 2–3, 11, 22, 30,
34, 42.
Illustrations: Lindsay Blow

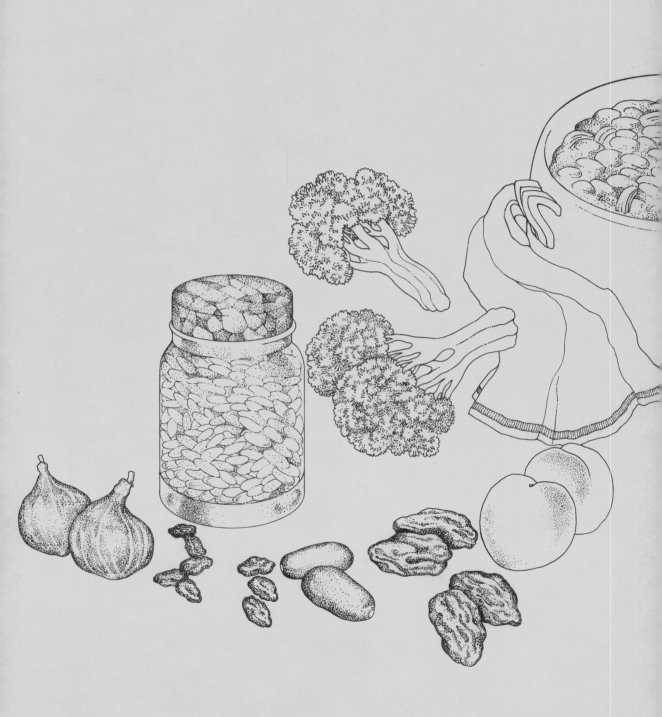